ERUPTION OF PERMANENT TEETH

A Color Atlas

Sadakatsu Sato, *D.D.S., D.Med.Sc.*

American Edition

Editor: Patricia Parsons, *D.M.D., M.S.*
Professor and chairman
Department of Pediatric Dentistry
Washington University
School of Dental Medicine

Ishiyaku EuroAmerica, Inc.
St. Louis · Tokyo

Translator: Bruce Talbot
Manuscript Editor: Joe Volpe

Ishiyaku EuroAmerica, Inc.
716 Hanley Industrial Court, St. Louis, Missouri 63144
1-44-2 Komagome, Toshima-ku, Tokyo 170, Japan

Library of Congress Catalogue Number 88-80817

Sato, Sadakatsu
    Eruption of Permanent Teeth

ISBN 0-912791-44-6

Ishiyaku EuroAmerica, Inc.
St. Louis · Tokyo

PREFACE

To gain an understanding of the eruption and occlusal formation of permanent teeth, dental researchers took maxillary and mandibular dental arch casts of a group of six-year-old children (initially 200 persons), at three-month intervals (i.e., four casts per year of each child), continuously for twelve years. However, it was found that taking casts at three-month intervals was not adequate for a full understanding of the eruption process.

Therefore, another study was undertaken in which sequential maxillary and mandibular casts were taken of children (initially 160) at two-month intervals, beginning at the age of eight months in order to follow the entire process, from the eruption and exfoliation of primary teeth to the eruption and occlusion of permanent teeth. This process included all of the mixed dentition stages.

These studies demonstrated that a shorter time interval was requisite for satisfactory observation of the progress of certain teeth — namely, the first and second molars. Factors such as the shape and eruption position of these teeth — even at the start of their eruption — have been shown to indicate adverse conditions that may eventually lead to dental caries.

The question regarding the particular forces involved in the eruption of primary and permanent teeth has already been discussed in detail in a variety of embryological studies. The purpose, however, of these studies has been to understand the kinds of forces involved in both the formation and occlusion of the teeth.

Children experiencing the eruption of primary or permanent teeth (up to the age of 11) generally fail to have an adequate grasp of dental hygiene. In addition, while their teeth have a relatively low resistance to caries, these children tend to have a relatively higher intake of sugar-laden foods. Research has shown that the saliva of such children serves as a more favorable environment than adult saliva for the growth of streptococcus mutans. In addition, among the permanent teeth, the first and second molars have the most complex occlusal surfaces and the deepest grooves and fissures. These factors promote the accumulation of food particles.

However, to understand the initial eruption process and the contamination conditions within the mouth, observations at two-month intervals did not suffice; the observation-interval was, therefore, shortened to one week. These weekly observations enabled us to understand in detail the amount of time elapsing between the confirmed start of tooth eruption to the completion of the eruption process, as well as the concomitant changes in the gingiva and the contamination of the occlusal surfaces that occur during this period. At the same time, it also enabled us to better understand the relation between the conditions of contamination and the occurrence of caries during eruption, which underscores the importance of preventive measures during this period. The primary concern of this study is the occurrence of caries during the eruption of permanent teeth, and especially during the early stages of first molar eruption.

It should also be noted that the first molars, popularly known as "six-year molars," because they are said to erupt during the child's sixth year, often erupt at age four or five. Several cases of first molar eruption in four-year-olds have been reported. In view of the above-mentioned factors present in children of this age — such as the inadequate grasp of proper tooth maintenance, the lower resistance to caries, and the molar's morphology, which is conducive to the accumulation of food particles — a detailed understanding of tooth contamination during the early stages of eruption is, therefore, an important and integral part of caries prevention.

This book is intended to be used by dental students, dental hygienists, and clinical dentists as an aid in the prevention of caries, by providing a detailed examination of occlusal surface eruption and the occurrence of dental caries.

I would like to thank Dr. Takashi Imada, chairman of Ishiyaku Publishers Co., for his editorial assistance and would also like to express my gratitude to Mr. Akira Morozumi, Dr. Masahiro Okamoto, Shuichi Yamaguchi and Katsuki Miyamoto for their cooperation in the compilation of the photographs and other materials.

Sadakatsu Sato, *D.D.S., D.Med.Sc.*
December 1985

CONTENTS

A Note on the Comparison of FDI and Japanese Formulas for Dentition

A) Deciduous Teeth

Japanese formula:

maxillary

$$\text{right} \quad \frac{\text{E D C B A} \ \vert \ \text{A B C D E}}{\text{E D C B A} \ \vert \ \text{A B C D E}} \quad \text{left}$$

mandibular

FDI formula:

maxillary

$$\text{right} \quad \begin{array}{c} 55 \ 54 \ 53 \ 52 \ 51 \quad 61 \ 62 \ 63 \ 64 \ 65 \\ 85 \ 84 \ 83 \ 82 \ 81 \quad 71 \ 72 \ 73 \ 74 \ 75 \end{array} \quad \text{left}$$

mandibular

Example comparisons:

$$\underline{D\vert} = 54$$
$$\overline{\vert C} = 73$$

B) Permanent Teeth

Japanese formula:

maxillary

$$\text{right} \quad \frac{8 \ 7 \ 6 \ 5 \ 4 \ 3 \ 2 \ 1 \ \vert \ 1 \ 2 \ 3 \ 4 \ 5 \ 6 \ 7 \ 8}{8 \ 7 \ 6 \ 5 \ 4 \ 3 \ 2 \ 1 \ \vert \ 1 \ 2 \ 3 \ 4 \ 5 \ 6 \ 7 \ 8} \quad \text{left}$$

mandibular

FDI formula:

maxillary

$$\text{right} \quad \begin{array}{c} 18 \ 17 \ 16 \ 15 \ 14 \ 13 \ 12 \ 11 \quad 21 \ 22 \ 23 \ 24 \ 25 \ 26 \ 27 \ 28 \\ 48 \ 47 \ 46 \ 45 \ 44 \ 43 \ 42 \ 41 \quad 31 \ 32 \ 33 \ 34 \ 35 \ 36 \ 37 \ 38 \end{array} \quad \text{left}$$

mandibular

Example comparisons:

$$\underline{4\vert} = 14$$
$$\overline{\vert 2} = 32$$
$$\overline{3\vert} = 43$$

Sequential Casts of the Same Child

(Record of every two months from 8 months to 15 years of age)

No. 199, Girl

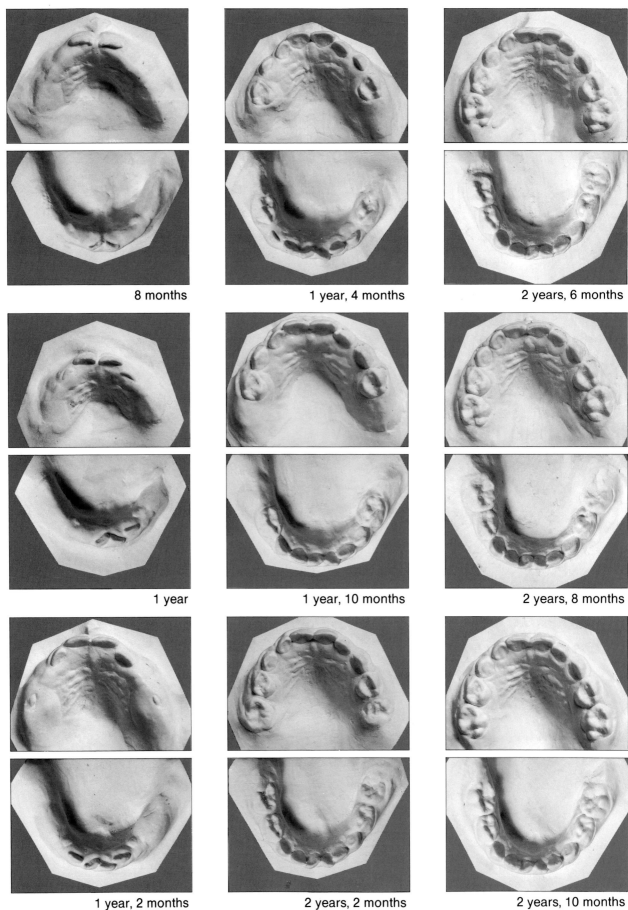

8 months	1 year, 4 months	2 years, 6 months
1 year	1 year, 10 months	2 years, 8 months
1 year, 2 months	2 years, 2 months	2 years, 10 months

I

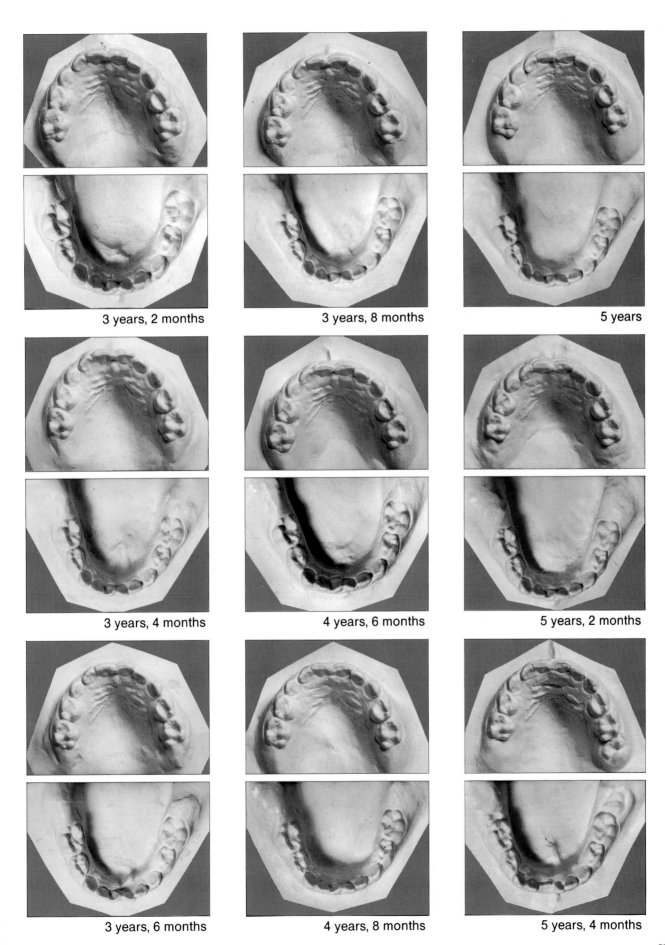

3 years, 2 months

3 years, 8 months

5 years

3 years, 4 months

4 years, 6 months

5 years, 2 months

3 years, 6 months

4 years, 8 months

5 years, 4 months

Sequential Casts of the Same Child

(Record of every two months from 8 months to 15 years of age)

No. 199, Girl

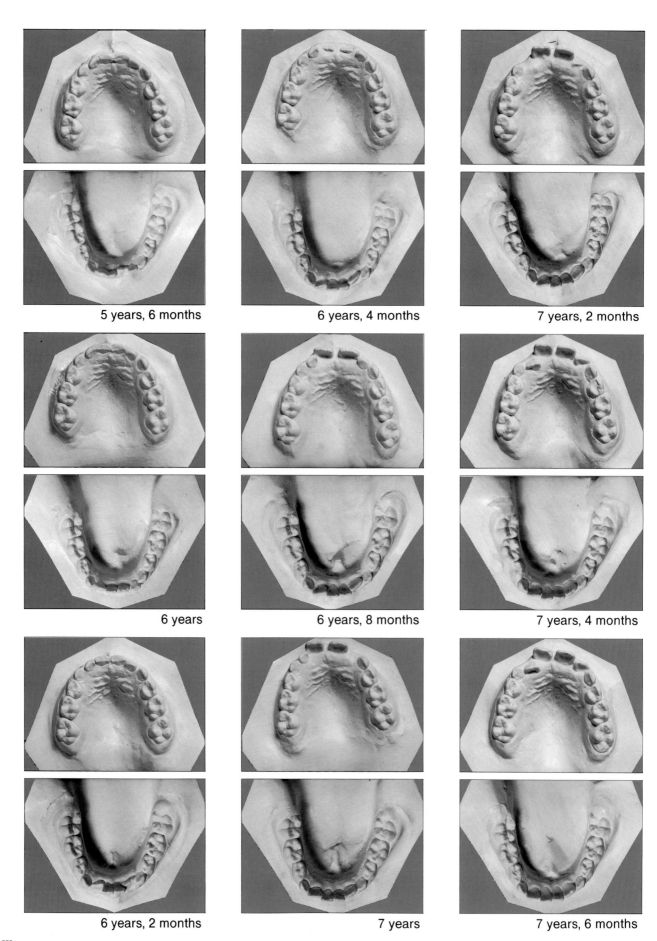

5 years, 6 months	6 years, 4 months	7 years, 2 months
6 years	6 years, 8 months	7 years, 4 months
6 years, 2 months	7 years	7 years, 6 months

III

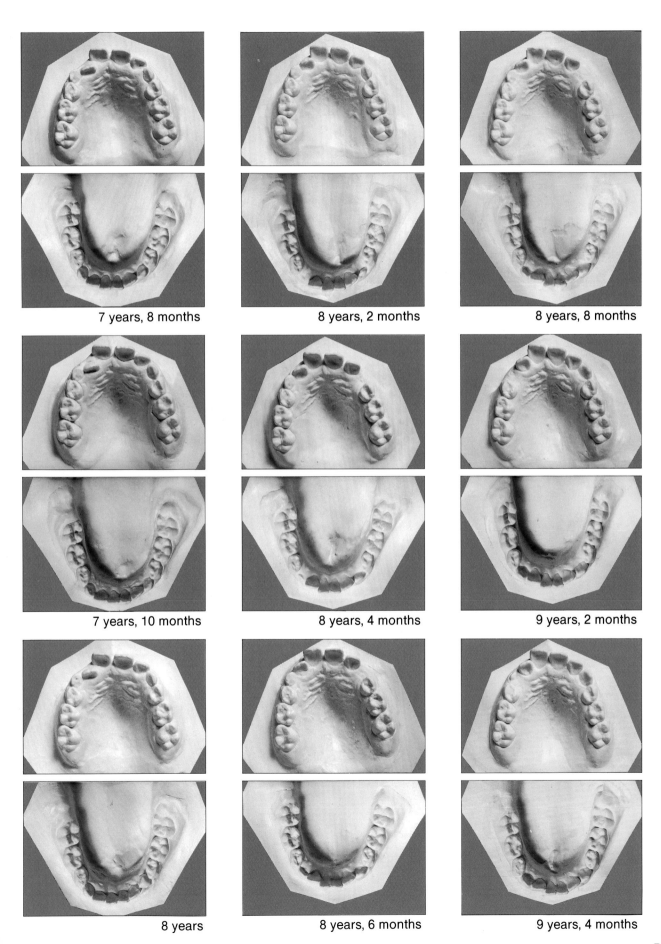

7 years, 8 months

8 years, 2 months

8 years, 8 months

7 years, 10 months

8 years, 4 months

9 years, 2 months

8 years

8 years, 6 months

9 years, 4 months

IV

Sequential Casts of the Same Child

(Record of every two months from 8 months to 15 years of age)

No. 199, Girl

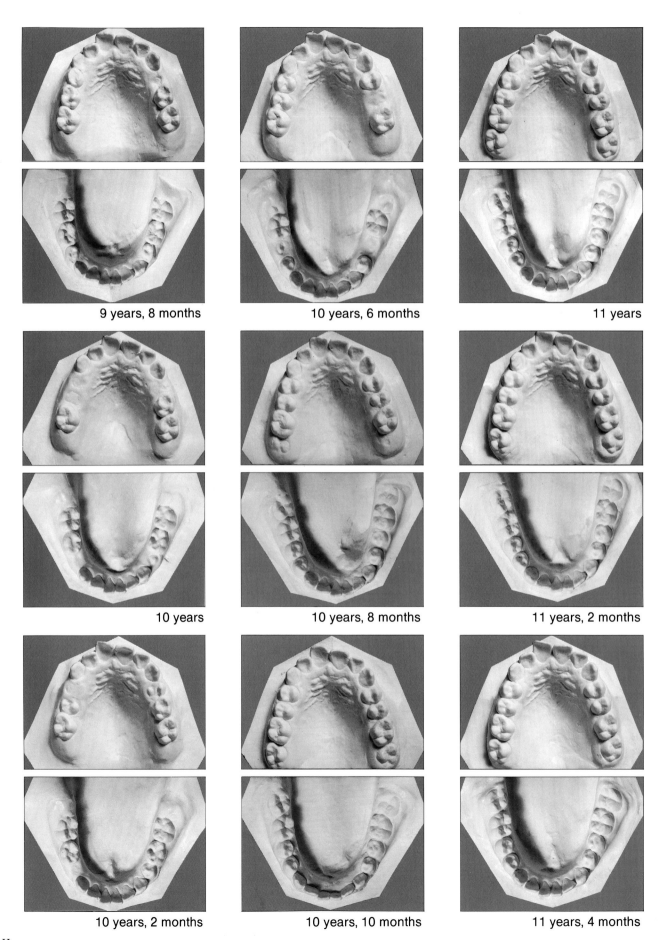

9 years, 8 months

10 years, 6 months

11 years

10 years

10 years, 8 months

11 years, 2 months

10 years, 2 months

10 years, 10 months

11 years, 4 months

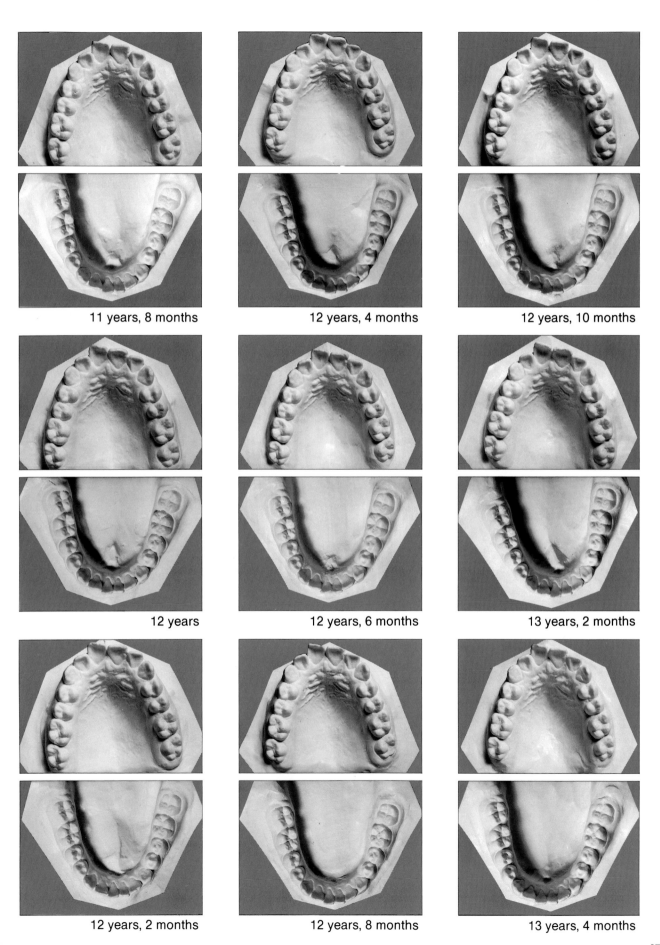

11 years, 8 months

12 years, 4 months

12 years, 10 months

12 years

12 years, 6 months

13 years, 2 months

12 years, 2 months

12 years, 8 months

13 years, 4 months

VI

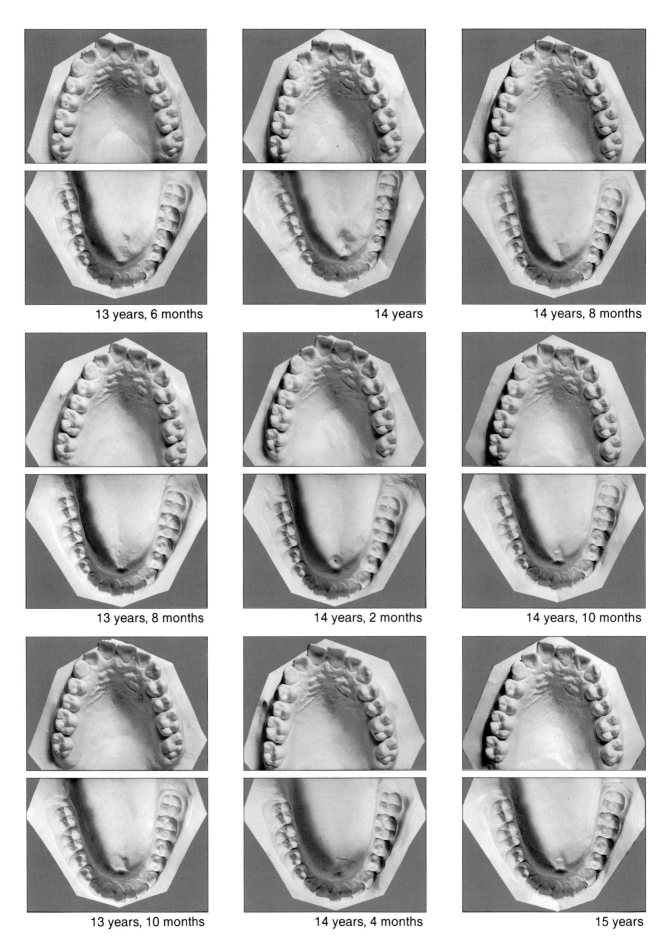

13 years, 6 months

14 years

14 years, 8 months

13 years, 8 months

14 years, 2 months

14 years, 10 months

13 years, 10 months

14 years, 4 months

15 years

SEQUENTIAL CASTS OF THE SAME CHILD

(Record of every two months)   No. 199, Girl

The plaster casts shown on the previous pages are sequential casts taken of the same child's maxillary and mandibular dental arches at two-month intervals, beginning at the age of 8 months and ending at 15 years. These casts were taken in order to trace the eruption of the primary and permanent teeth and their occlusal development.

Initially, 160 children took part in this project. This number grew to over 600 as the project continued. The example shown here is just one of the hundreds of subjects involved.

Primary Dentition Period (No. 199)

The maxillary and mandibular primary molars began erupting at 8 months of age and by 2 years and 2 months, all of the primary teeth had erupted. All of the primary teeth were very healthy, with no sign of caries during their entire period in the dental arch.

The primary dental arch showed normal occlusion; however, there was a slight primate gap in the maxillary and mandibular arches that continued until age four. There were no gaps between any of the other teeth. The primary dentition remained intact until age 5 years, 2 months, when replacement by permanent teeth (the mixed dentition period) began. A vertical-type relation existed between the distal sides of the maxillary and mandibular primary second molars (the terminal plane).

Permanent Dentition
(Eruption of Occlusal Surfaces)

The first of the four permanent first molars began erupting when the child was 5 years and 2 months old. The eruption was foreshadowed by gingival swelling on the distal side of the mandibular left and right primary second molars.

At 5 years, 4 months: 6|, |6 and |6 begin to erupt. The mesiobuccal, mesiolingual, and buccal cusps of |6 appear, as far as the mesial small grooves and the central sulcus on the occlusal surface. As 6| erupts, its mesiobuccal and mesiolingual cusps appear, and, as |6 erupts, its mesiobuccal, mesiolingual, and lingual cusps emerge as far as the mesial small grooves on the occlusal surface. A| has exfoliated. 1| also begins to erupt at this time, and emerges to the central edge.

At 5 years, 6 months (2 months after the start of eruption):   As for 6|, |6 and |6, most of the occlusal surfaces have erupted, although a small amount of the tissue remains on the distal edge. Although there was no sign of 6| erupting two months earlier, by this time most of its occlusal surface has erupted and only its distal edge remains covered by tissue. At 5 years and 8 months, |A has exfoliated. |1 also begins to erupt at this time, while 1| has already completely erupted.

At 6 years (6 months after the start of eruption):   The occlusal surfaces of 6| and |6 have erupted completely, while the distal edges of 6| and |6 remain covered by tissue.

At 6 years, 2 months: B| and |B have exfoliated while 2| and |2 have begun to erupt and rotate lingually.

At 6 years, 4 months: A| and |A have exfoliated while 1| and |1 have begun to erupt, emerging as far as the

central to mesial edges. The entire incisal edges of 2| and |2 have erupted completely by this time.

At 6 years, 6 months: The occlusal surfaces of 6| and |6 have not yet erupted completely. The incisal edges of 1| and |1 have erupted completely.

At 7 years: The occlusal surfaces of 6| and |6 have erupted, although one can still see tissue on the distal margin, after an eruption period of nearly 1 year and 8 months. |B has exfoliated.

At 7 years, 2 months: |2 begins to erupt and B| has exfoliated.

At 7 years, 4 months: The incisal edges of 2| and |2 have erupted completely, and these teeth are rotating toward the palate.

At 8 years, 2 months: C| and |C have exfoliated and |3 has begun to erupt.

At 8 years, 4 months: 3| has begun to erupt and |C has exfoliated.

At 8 years, 6 months: |3 has erupted completely.

At 8 years, 8 months: 3| has erupted completely.

At 8 years, 10 months: |3 has begun to erupt.

At 9 years: C| has exfoliated. |3 has begun to erupt.

At 9 years, 2 months: The incisal edge of |3 has erupted completely.

At 9 years, 4 months: 3| has begun to erupt.

At 9 years, 8 months: |D has exfoliated.

At 9 years, 10 months: |D has exfoliated.

At 10 years: The bucccal cusps of |4 and |4 have begun to erupt. The incisal edge of 3| has erupted completely. E|, D|, and |D have exfoliated.

At 10 years, 2 months: |4 has begun erupting as the lingual cusps emerge (as far as nearly one-third of the occlusal surface). 5| has erupted as far as nearly four-fifths of the occlusal surface. The occlusal surface of |4 has erupted completely. 4| has begun to erupt. |7 has begun to erupt from the mesiobuccal cusp.

At 10 years, 6 months: The occlusal surfaces of 5| and |4 have begun to erupt. Most of the occlusal surface of |4 has erupted. 5| begins to erupt from the buccal cusps. |E and |E have exfoliated and 5| and 4| have begun to erupt. |7 has begun to erupt from the mesiobuccal cusps. |7 has begun to erupt as the mesiolingual cusp emerges to the mesial groove.

At 10 years, 8 months: 7| and |7 have begun to erupt. The occlusal surface of 4| has erupted completely. Most of the occlusal surface of |5 has erupted. The mesial, distal, and lingual cusps of 7| and |7 have erupted and about three-quarters of the occlusal surfaces have emerged. Most of the occlusal surface of |5 has emerged (gaps are visible around this tooth).

At 10 years, 10 months: The occlusal surface of |5 has erupted completely. The occlusal surfaces of 7| and |7 are about four-fifths erupted. The occlusal surfaces of 7| and |7 are about four-fifths erupted. The occlusal surfaces of |5 and |5 have erupted completely.

At 11 years, 2 months: The occlusal surfaces of 7| and |7 have erupted completely. The distal edges of 7| and |7 have not yet erupted completely.

At 11 years, 4 months: The occlusal surfaces of 7| and |7 have erupted completely. The full eruption of the occlusal surfaces of the second molars required from 6 months to 1 year and 2 months.

SEQUENTIAL CASTS OF THE SAME CHILD
Phases of Occlusion

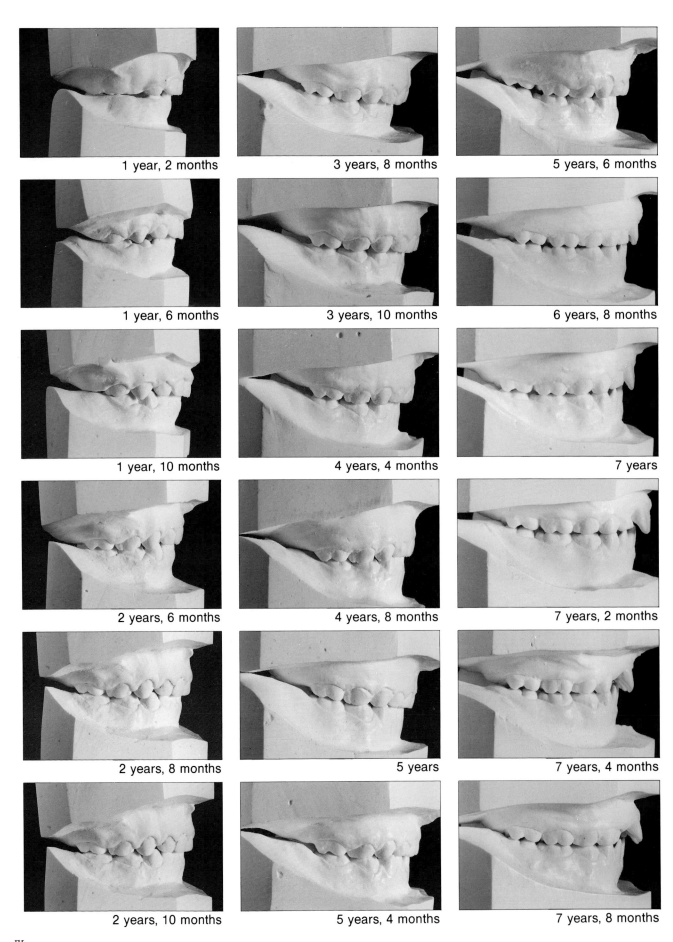

1 year, 2 months

3 years, 8 months

5 years, 6 months

1 year, 6 months

3 years, 10 months

6 years, 8 months

1 year, 10 months

4 years, 4 months

7 years

2 years, 6 months

4 years, 8 months

7 years, 2 months

2 years, 8 months

5 years

7 years, 4 months

2 years, 10 months

5 years, 4 months

7 years, 8 months

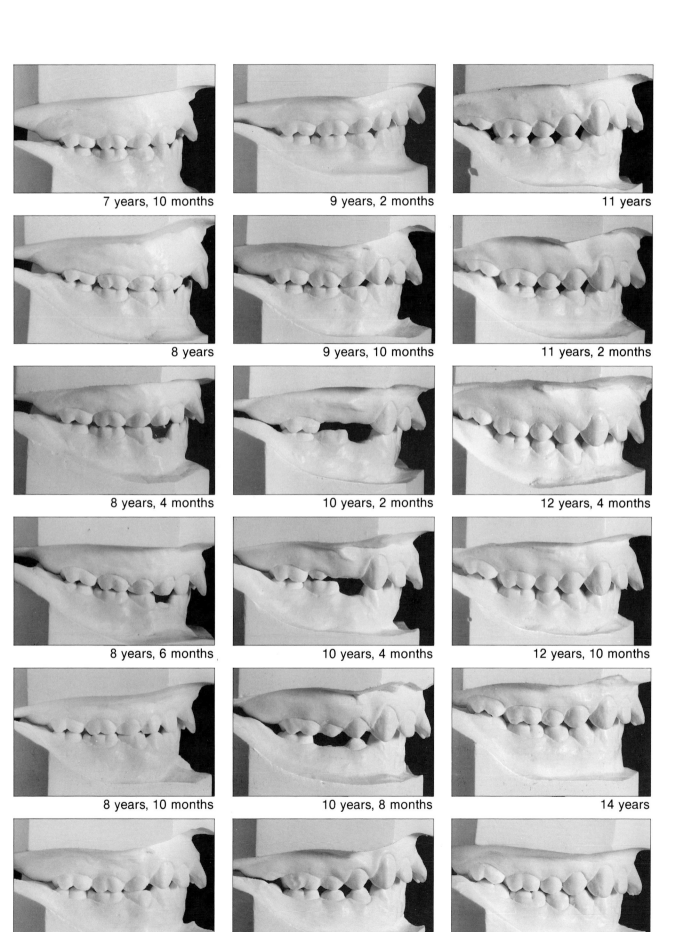

7 years, 10 months

9 years, 2 months

11 years

8 years

9 years, 10 months

11 years, 2 months

8 years, 4 months

10 years, 2 months

12 years, 4 months

8 years, 6 months

10 years, 4 months

12 years, 10 months

8 years, 10 months

10 years, 8 months

14 years

9 years

10 years, 10 months

15 years

X

SEQUENTIAL CASTS OF THE SAME CHILD

Phases of Occlusion

Occlusion of Primary Teeth

Initial occlusion begins with the eruption of the primary first molar. Although the primary central and lateral incisors erupt at around 8 months of age, their role is not so much to occlude, for mastication, but to bite and tear food. Development of the occlusion of the primary teeth continues until about age 5, as the full primary dentition completes its eruption. At this stage, the eruption of permanent teeth begins.

Occlusion of Permanent Teeth

Occlusion of permanent teeth began with the exchange of primary teeth (the mixed dentition period). This occlusion was preceded by resorption of the primary roots which led to a loosening of the primary teeth and a reduction in occlusal force. To compensate for this reduction, the first permanent molars erupted behind the primary second molars and thus began the occlusion of the permanent teeth.

At 5 years and 4 months, first molars emerged on the maxillary left and mandibular left and right sides, and two months later, the maxillary right first molar began to erupt. Their occlusion was not yet complete, however, and the primary teeth were still relied upon almost entirely to perform mastication. At about the same time, the mandibular right central incisor began to erupt. This tooth erupted completely between ages 6 years and 8 months and 7 years. Occlusion of the first molars required from 1 year and 6 months to 1 year and 8 months altogether. By age 7, all mandibular incisors erupted. However, the occlusion at this point was end-to-end and had not yet become either a vertical type or a Class I distal type.

At 5 years and 8 months, $\overline{1|}$ began to erupt, and $\overline{1|1}$ both reached the occlusal line 6 months later, at 6 years and 2 months. Once the first molars had erupted, exchange of the incisal teeth began. After the mandibular central and lateral incisors had erupted, the maxillary central and lateral incisor started erupting (beginning at 5 years and 4 months). Each of the incisors required from 7 to 8 months to reach the occlusal line, and by the age of 8 all had reached this line.

From about age 9 to age 10, the primary canines and primary first and second molars began to exfoliate. In all four quadrants, these teeth fell out either simultaneously or in close succession. Accordingly, this period is one of difficult mastication using the primary teeth, a condition that soon improves when the first molars reach the occlusal line (see the photos titled 10 years, 2 months to 10 years, 10 months).

In this example (No. 199), at 8 years and 2 months, $\overline{C|C}$ fell out and $\overline{3}$ erupted. At 8 years and 4 months, $3|$ erupted and $|C$ fell out.

At 8 years and 10 months, $|3$ erupted and, at 9 years and 2 months, $C|$ fell out. At 9 years and 4 months, $3|$ erupted, but the maxillary and mandibular canines still had not reached full occlusion. $|D$ exfoliated at 9 years and 8 months and $\overline{|D}$ at 9 years and 10 months. At 10 years, $\underline{ED|}$ and $\overline{D|}$ exfoliated and $|4$ and $\overline{|4}$ began to erupt.

At 10 years and 2 months, $\underline{5|}$ and $\underline{4|}$ began to erupt, but as can be seen in the photographs, in the lateral section only the first molars are occluding. This condition continued for a period of almost two years until, at about age 11, the second premolars erupted and occluded.

At about 10 years and 2 months, $\overline{7|}$ began to erupt, and $\underline{7|}$, $\underline{|7}$, and $\overline{7|}$ erupted six months later, at 10 years and 8 months, The second molars, however, had still not reached the occlusal line. They finally reached the occlusal line at age 11 years and 8 months, and thus their occlusion required a period of 6 months to 1 year and 2 months.

Part I INTRODUCTION

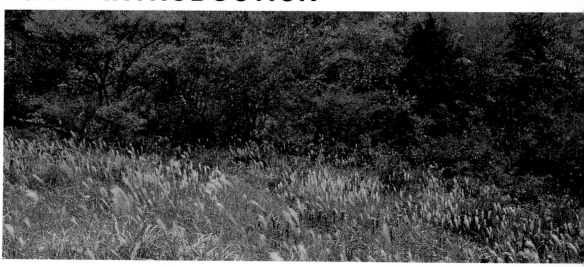

1 ⟋ TOOTH ERUPTION

The term "tooth eruption" generally refers to the appearance of some part of a tooth above the surface of the gingiva. However, eruption actually includes the entire embryological process from the formation of the tooth germs, in the mandible and maxilla, to calcification, crown formation, and root formation. The root is only about one-third formed when the crown begins to erupt into the oral cavity. Not only is this embryological process part of eruption, but so is the long process of occlusal development. Thus, the emergence of teeth into the oral cavity is only one part of the total eruption process.

If we use this broad definition of the eruption process in observing eruption periods, it becomes apparent that just about any of the periods can be interpreted as part of the eruption process. This means, for example, that various observational studies of tooth age, based on eruption times as their point of reference, are likely to employ non-uniform points of reference. Therefore, some standard point of reference must be determined so as to ensure uniformity among academic and clinical observational studies. For lack of an established standard, we have chosen to help ensure at least a relative uniformity by dividing observational studies into those which use a broad definition of eruption and those which use the narrow definition—namely the first appearance of a tooth above the gingival surface.

1) Embryological Tooth Eruption

Embryological tooth eruption is the process commencing with tooth germ formation and ending with eruption of the tooth into the oral cavity. This term is relatively easy to understand in the context of the broad definition of eruption, i.e. the process including everything from tooth germ formation to complete occlusion.

2) Clinical Tooth Eruption

Clinical tooth eruption refers to the appearance of some part of the tooth above the gingival surface (defined as the "beginning of eruption" or the "eruption time"). Eruption-time surveys commonly employ a number of different survey methods. Most of these methods draw a close parallel between dental growth and development and overall physical growth and development, as evidenced in the commonly used term "six-year molars" for first molars, a term which directly links these molars' eruption to a particular year in the child's development.

3) Time of Clinical Tooth Eruption

The time of clinical tooth eruption (a tooth's appearance in the oral cavity) was described by L. M. Carr as the time when the tooth breaks through the gingiva and part of the tooth can be observed. This definition of tooth eruption time can be adopted as a standard survey method to enable uniform eruption time observations.

NOTE: Hereafter, the clinical interpretation of eruption will be employed and all discussion of eruption start times will be according to Carr's method.

4) Eruption Of Occlusal Surfaces And Completion Of Eruption

Eruption begins with the incisal edges of the incisors, the cusp tips, and then the mesial and distal corners of the canines. It also begins with the buccal and lingual cusps to the mesial and distal marginal ridges of the molars. Eruption of all of these teeth is completed by the emergence of their edges and occlusal surfaces (see Figs. 1, 2, 3, 4, and 5).

2 CHARACTERISTICS OF ERUPTION

1) Incisors

The incisors have sharply tapered crowns suitable for the cutting and tearing of food. The alignment of the incisors affects both facial appearance and pronunciation.

The hardening of the incisors begins with the front edge, in other words, the incisal edge or peak, and their calcification begins from the central incisal tubercle and advances along the incisal edge, progressing mesially and distally. Eruption begins following calcification.

The incisor (maxillary central and lateral incisors and mandibular central and lateral incisors) erupt from their incisal edges and have a sharp, flat crown that is conducive to relatively rapid eruption.

The primary incisors are replaced after the eruption of the permanent first molars, and the mandibular and maxillary central incisors all erupt rapidly. Together with the first molars, they play an important part in the formation of the permanent dental arch. There are times, however, when the incisors erupt before the molars.

2) Canines

The canines erupt at the cusp tip and exhibit a spear-like shape.

3) Molars

The molars include the premolars and the molars, two types which differ both in function and in anatomical form.

a) Premolars
The premolars include the first and second premolars in all four quadrants. However, the maxillary and mandibular premolars have different occlusal surface shapes. While the maxillary first and second premolars have nearly identical occlusal surfaces, those of the mandibular first and second premolars are different.

The maxillary first and second premolars have both the buccal and lingual cusps. The buccal cusp, like that of the molar, has a well developed peak. The lingual cusp is also relatively well developed.

The mandibular first premolars have a well developed buccal cusp but a relatively poorly defined lingual cusp. The mandibular second premolars have almost equally developed buccal and lingual cusps. For the first and second premolars, the buccal cusp is usually the first to erupt.

b) Molars
The molars include first and second molars in all four quadrants. They all have many functional and anatomical features in common, although some features are different.

As for the first molars, the maxillary first molars have four cusps, while the mandibular first molars have five and a larger occlusal surface. The first molars erupt behind the primary second molars. The first molars normally erupt in this position. They are known as the key to the formation of the permanent dental arch, and they have the strongest occlusive force.

As for the second molars, the maxillary and mandibular second molars both have four cusps. However, the maxillary second molars have a degenerative tendency and sometimes appear with only three cusps or with an overall stunted anatomical form.

In the second molars, the mesiobuccal cusp is usually the first to emerge, followed by the mesiolingual cusp, the distobuccal cusp, and the distolingual cusp — in that order. Only the mandibular first molars have five cusps, and their distobuccal cusp is the last to erupt. This eruption order is the same as the ontogenetic order of cusp formation.

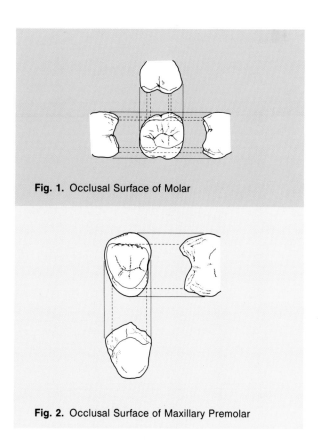

Fig. 1. Occlusal Surface of Molar

Fig. 2. Occlusal Surface of Maxillary Premolar

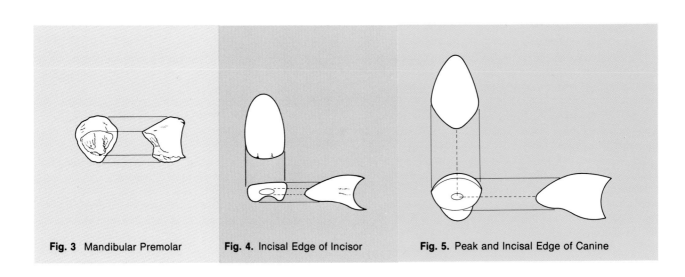

Fig. 3 Mandibular Premolar   **Fig. 4.** Incisal Edge of Incisor   **Fig. 5.** Peak and Incisal Edge of Canine

Tooth Type / Stage	Eruption Stage	Incisor	Canine	Eruption Stage	Molar
I		Part of central incisal edge	Part of peak		Part of mesio-buccal and lingual cusps
II		Part of mesial edge and corner	Part of mesial and distal edges		Mesiolingual cusp and mesial edge
III		Part of the distal edge and corner	Part of mesial and distal corners		One third to two thirds of occlusal surface including part of central groove
IV		Entire incisor	Entire canine including the mesial and distal corners		About two thirds of occlusal surface including the central and distal grooves
V					Entire molar including distal edge

Fig. 6. Occlusal Surface Eruption Stages of Various Teeth

(Source: Sato)

Eruption time for permanent teeth vary widely from one person to the next. The development process, in which primary teeth are exchanged for permanent teeth, is a physiological phenomenon having characteristics not seen in any other body organ. The exfoliation of primary teeth and the subsequent eruption of permanent teeth is a developmental phenomenon that forms part of the body's continual process of growth.

1) Systemic Factors

If the body's overall development is advanced, the permanent teeth erupt earlier than usual. If this development is retarded, tooth eruption comes later. In Japan, studies relating permanent tooth eruption to body height and weight were conducted in 1955 and 1982. The 1982 study showed, for certain permanent teeth, an average eruption age a whole year earlier than that of the 1955 study. This discrepancy is thought to be due to systemic factors, i.e. a modern trend toward earlier overall development (see Tables 2 and 3 and Fig. 7).

2) Local Factors

The eruption of teeth is defined as the appearance of teeth in the oral cavity, and the time of eruption is expressed in terms of the individual's age (hence the expression "eruption age") (see Table 1).

With the exception of the permanent molars, permanent teeth are often influenced by their primary predecessors. Disturbances in primary teeth (such as caries) often lead to abnormal root resorption, which in turn delays or otherwise disturbs the eruption of permanent teeth. If primary teeth exfoliate prematurely, the permanent successors sometimes erupt prematurely, or can even be delayed in erupting due to a hardening of the gingiva.

Table 1. Eruption Times of Permanent Teeth

		Maxillary		Mandibular	
		Average Age	Standard Variation	Average Age	Standard Variation
Central Incisors	Boy	7. 11	0. 86	6. 33	0. 59
	Girl	7. 02	0. 78	6. 13	0. 41
Lateral Incisors	Boy	8. 25	0. 66	7. 21	0. 78
	Girl	7. 97	0. 78	6. 95	0. 66
Canines	Boy	10. 69	0. 86	10. 04	1. 06
	Girl	10. 28	0. 93	9. 27	0. 90
First Premolars	Boy	10. 06	1. 21	9. 87	1. 36
	Girl	10. 01	1. 04	9. 58	1. 18
Second Premolars	Boy	10. 65	1. 34	10. 05	1. 26
	Girl	10. 57	1. 16	10. 34	1. 15
First Molars	Boy	6. 59	0. 76	6. 29	0. 75
	Girl	6. 36	0. 61	6. 04	0. 63
Second Molars	Boy	11. 91	0. 80	11. 55	0. 74
	Girl	11. 95	0. 93	11. 45	0. 77

(Source: Sato Institute of Dental Research)

Table 2. Height and Weight at Permanent Teeth Eruption Times

		Height (cm)		Weight (kg)	
		Boy	Girl	Boy	Girl
Maxillary	Central Incisors	113.7cm	112.5cm	20.16kg	19.59kg
	Lateral Incisors	120.7	119.0	22.72	21.41
	Canines	132.7	131.2	29.55	26.97
	First Premolars	127.8	126.3	27.94	26.20
	Second Premolars	133.3	132.8	31.58	29.87
	First Molars	111.6	110.5		
	Second Molars	141.2	139.4	34.71	32.86
Mandibular	Central Incisors	110.5	109.4	19.59	18.07
	Lateral Incisors	114.4	113.4	20.96	19.71
	Canines	130.0	123.4	28.08	24.35
	First Premolars	123.6	127.9	28.73	26.60
	Second Premolars	133.5	133.4	31.55	29.35
	First Molars	110.1	109.8		
	Second Molars	140.4	139.8	32.75	30.76

(Source: Sato Institute of Dental Research)

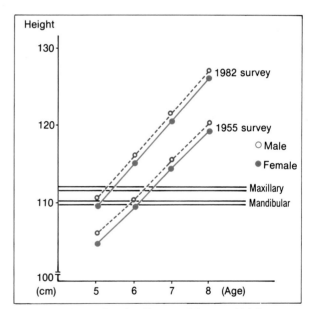

Fig. 7. First Molar Eruption Times and Average Height
(Comparison of 1955 and 1982 Surveys)

(Source: Japanese Ministry of Education)

Table 3. Comparison of Height and Age of Boys and Girls at First Molar Eruption Time　　　(Height unit: cm)

	Boys				Girls			
Age	5 yrs.	6 yrs.	7 yrs.	8 yrs.	5 yrs.	6 yrs.	7 yrs.	8 yrs.
1955	106.0	110.3	115.6	120.3	104.9	109.3	114.6	119.4
1982	110.4	115.9	121.5	127.0	109.6	115.2	120.8	126.3
Differential	4.4	5.6	5.9	6.7	4.7	5.9	6.2	6.9

(Source: Japanese Ministry of Education)

The eruption order of permanent teeth is a major factor in the formation and occlusion of the permanent dental arch. The permanent dental arch is formed as a product of the eruption of a total of 32 permanent teeth from the maxillary and mandibular jaws. The order and positions in which tooth No. 1 to tooth No. 32 erupt comprise the body's physiological mechanism for the growth and development of occlusion and mastication.

Consider, for example, the popular name for first molars: "six-year molars." The name conveys the impression that these molars erupt as a result of the child's reaching the age of six. However, the actual causes are much more complex: around this age, the roots of the anterior primary teeth begin to resorb, resulting in the primary teeth's exfoliation and a corresponding decline in the dental arch's occlusal force. In response to the need for greater occlusal force, the first molars erupt behind the primary dental arch. Fittingly, the first molars are not as prone as other permanent teeth to being influenced by disturbances in the primary teeth, and this helps them to erupt in a normal position with relative ease and to play their key role as the trail blazer and leader of the permanent dental arch.

Although the most accurate method for studying eruption order (and positions) of permanent teeth is to trace the dental history of the same individual, many researchers, in consideration of the many years and the various difficulties involved in this method, have opted to study this order in terms of average eruption times (average age at time of eruption).

1) Separate Eruption Orders of Maxillary and Mandibular Teeth

The eruption order of teeth is usually discussed separately for maxillary and mandibular teeth and for right and left sides. In Table 4, we see 21 different maxillary eruption orders and 22 different mandibular eruption orders among a large number of individuals surveyed. We can also note that eruption orders 1 and 2 (for both jaws) are typical among the Japanese (see Table 4).

2) Overall Eruption Order

The maxillary and mandibular permanent teeth progress toward the occlusal line as they erupt. There is no generally valid description of the order of tooth eruption, nor do the teeth erupt in a simple and predictable pattern, since they are easily influenced by individual differences, including such factors as disturbances in eruption, hereditary characteristics, and environmental factors.

Out of the 373 individuals observed every three months over a period of 12 years, eruption order predictions proved inaccurate in 259 cases (see Table 5 and Fig. 7).

The most frequent eruption order among the cases surveyed was: $\overline{6} \rightarrow \underline{6} \rightarrow \overline{1} \rightarrow \underline{1} \rightarrow \overline{2} \rightarrow \underline{2} \rightarrow \overline{3} \rightarrow \overline{4} \rightarrow \underline{4} \rightarrow \underline{3} \rightarrow \overline{5} \rightarrow \underline{5} \rightarrow \overline{7} \rightarrow \underline{7}$. Note, however, that this most frequent order occurred in

Table 4. Eruption Order of Permanent Teeth   (For Each Jaw)

Eruption Order No.	Maxillary — Eruption Order							Maxillary %	Mandibular — Eruption Order							Mandibular %
1	6	1	2	4	3	5	7	50.4	6	1	2	3	4	5	7	56.6
2	6	1	2	3	4	5	7	21.4	6	1	2	3	4	7	5	13.4
3	6	1	2	4	5	3	7	12.1	6	1	2	4	3	5	7	10.5
4	6	1	2	4	3	7	5	4.3	1	6	2	3	4	5	7	4.0
5	6	1	2	3	4	7	5	2.9	6	1	2	3	7	4	5	3.8
6	6	1	2	4	7	3	5	1.6	6	1	2	3	5	4	7	1.9
7	6	1	2	4	5	7	3	0.8	6	1	2	4	3	7	5	1.6
8	1	2	6	4	3	5	7	0.8	6	1	2	7	3	4	5	1.6
9	1	6	2	3	4	5	7	0.8	6	1	2	4	5	3	7	1.1
10	6	1	2	3	7	4	5	0.5	6	1	2	5	4	3	7	1.1
11	6	1	2	5	4	3	7	0.5	6	1	2	5	3	4	7	0.8
12	6	1	2	7	3	5	4	0.5	6	1	2	3	7	5	4	0.5
13	6	1	4	2	3	5	7	0.5	6	1	2	4	7	3	5	0.5
14	6	1	4	2	5	3	7	0.5	1	6	2	3	4	7	5	0.5
15	1	2	6	4	5	3	7	0.5	6	1	2	3	5	7	4	0.3
16	6	1	2	4	7	5	3	0.3	6	1	2	7	4	3	5	0.3
17	6	1	2	7	4	5	3	0.3	1	6	2	7	4	5	3	0.3
18	6	1	4	2	5	7	3	0.3	6	1	2	3	7	4	5	0.3
19	6	4	1	2	5	3	7	0.3	1	6	2	4	3	7	5	0.3
20	1	2	6	3	4	5	7	0.3	1	6	2	7	3	4	5	0.3
21	1	6	2	4	3	5	7	0.3	1	2	6	3	4	5	7	0.3
22									6	1	4	2	5	3	7	0.3

(Source: Haruhiko Kitamura)

only 2.53% of the cases, and that all other eruption orders occurred in less than 2.0% of the cases.

One of the major reasons for this great diversity in overall eruption orders is the wide variation in the eruption order of the maxillary and mandibular lateral teeth, which generally erupt in close succession, and the tendency of the second molar to erupt even earlier than the second premolar.

Even though the overall eruption order is complex and unpredictable, it is easier to understand if we look at the eruption times of individual teeth. For example, we can see in Table 6 that there is a high probability that the three teeth, 6, 1, and 2, will erupt in that order. Accordingly, in clinical practice, we can monitor the eruption times of these three teeth with reference to the age and developmental figures in the table. Likewise, in monitoring the eruption times of the lateral teeth, we should note such factors as the relationship between maxillary and mandibular lateral teeth and should consider eruption-promoting measures for these teeth if a disturbancer in their primary predecessors has been confirmed (see Tables 6, 7, and 8 and Figs. 8 and 9).

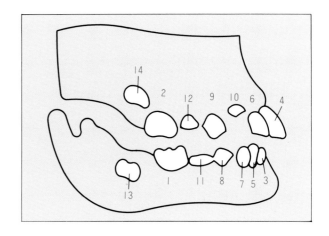

Table 5. Eruption Order of Both Jaws

Eruption Order No.	Eruption Order 1	2	3	4	5	6	7	8	9	10	11	12	13	14	No. of Cases 373	%
1	$\overline{6}$	$\underline{6}$	$\overline{1}$	$\underline{1}$	$\overline{2}$	$\underline{2}$	$\overline{3}$	$\overline{4}$	$\underline{4}$	$\underline{3}$	$\overline{5}$	$\underline{5}$	$\overline{7}$	$\underline{7}$	9	2.53
2							$\overline{3}$	$\underline{4}$	$\underline{3}$	$\overline{4}$	$\overline{5}$	$\underline{5}$	$\overline{7}$	$\underline{7}$	7	1.97
3							$\overline{3}$	$\overline{4}$	$\underline{4}$	$\underline{3}$	$\overline{5}$	$\underline{5}$	$\overline{7}$	$\underline{7}$	6	1.69
134	$\overline{6}$	$\underline{6}$	$\overline{1}$	$\underline{1}$	$\overline{2}$	$\underline{4}$	$\underline{2}$	$\overline{3}$	$\overline{4}$	$\underline{5}$	$\underline{5}$	$\underline{3}$	$\overline{7}$	$\overline{7}$	2	0.56
135							$\underline{2}$	$\overline{3}$	$\overline{4}$	$\underline{3}$	$\overline{5}$	$\underline{6}$	$\overline{7}$	$\underline{7}$	1	0.28
136							$\underline{2}$	$\overline{4}$	$\overline{3}$	$\underline{4}$	$\underline{5}$	$\overline{7}$	$\underline{5}$	$\overline{7}$	1	0.28
137							$\underline{2}$	$\overline{3}$	$\underline{3}$	$\underline{5}$	$\overline{4}$	$\underline{5}$	$\overline{7}$	$\underline{7}$	1	0.28
138							$\underline{2}$	$\overline{3}$	$\overline{3}$	$\underline{5}$	$\overline{4}$	$\underline{5}$	$\overline{7}$	$\underline{7}$	1	0.28
140	$\overline{6}$	$\underline{6}$	$\overline{1}$	$\underline{1}$	$\overline{2}$	$\underline{4}$	$\underline{2}$	$\overline{3}$	$\overline{4}$	$\underline{3}$	$\underline{5}$	$\overline{5}$	$\overline{7}$	$\underline{7}$	1	0.28
141							$\underline{2}$	$\overline{3}$	$\underline{3}$	$\overline{4}$	$\underline{5}$	$\underline{5}$	$\overline{7}$	$\underline{7}$	1	0.28
142							$\underline{2}$	$\overline{4}$	$\underline{3}$	$\underline{5}$	$\overline{3}$	$\underline{5}$	$\overline{7}$	$\underline{7}$	1	0.28
143							$\underline{2}$	$\overline{5}$	$\underline{4}$	$\overline{3}$	$\underline{3}$	$\underline{5}$	$\overline{7}$	$\underline{7}$	1	0.28
144							$\underline{2}$	$\overline{3}$	$\overline{5}$	$\underline{3}$	$\underline{4}$	$\overline{7}$	$\underline{5}$	$\overline{7}$	1	0.28
145							$\overline{3}$	$\underline{2}$	$\underline{4}$	$\underline{3}$	$\overline{5}$	$\underline{5}$	$\overline{7}$	$\underline{7}$	1	0.28
146	$\overline{6}$	$\underline{6}$	$\overline{1}$	$\underline{1}$	$\overline{2}$	$\overline{3}$	$\underline{2}$	$\overline{4}$	$\underline{3}$	$\overline{4}$	$\overline{7}$	$\underline{7}$	$\overline{5}$	$\underline{5}$	1	0.28
147							$\overline{4}$	$\underline{2}$	$\overline{4}$	$\underline{5}$	$\overline{7}$	$\underline{3}$	$\underline{5}$	$\overline{7}$	1	0.28
148	$\overline{6}$	$\underline{6}$	$\overline{1}$	$\underline{1}$	$\overline{2}$	$\underline{2}$	$\overline{3}$	$\overline{7}$	$\underline{4}$	$\overline{4}$	$\underline{3}$	$\overline{7}$	$\underline{5}$	$\underline{5}$	1	0.28
149							$\underline{4}$	$\overline{3}$	$\overline{4}$	$\underline{3}$	$\underline{5}$	$\overline{7}$	$\underline{5}$	$\overline{7}$	1	0.28
150							$\underline{4}$	$\overline{4}$	$\underline{3}$	$\overline{3}$	$\overline{5}$	$\underline{5}$	$\overline{7}$	$\underline{7}$	1	0.28
151	$\overline{6}$	$\underline{6}$	$\overline{1}$	$\underline{1}$	$\overline{2}$	$\overline{5}$	$\underline{2}$	$\overline{4}$	$\underline{3}$	$\overline{4}$	$\underline{3}$	$\underline{5}$	$\overline{7}$	$\underline{7}$	1	0.28
152	$\overline{6}$	$\underline{6}$	$\overline{1}$	$\underline{1}$	$\overline{4}$	$\overline{2}$	$\overline{3}$	$\underline{2}$	$\underline{4}$	$\overline{5}$	$\underline{3}$	$\underline{5}$	$\overline{7}$	$\underline{7}$	1	0.28
153	$\overline{6}$	$\underline{6}$	$\overline{1}$	1	$\overline{4}$	$\underline{2}$	$\overline{2}$	$\overline{3}$	$\underline{4}$	$\overline{5}$	$\underline{3}$	$\underline{5}$	$\overline{7}$	$\underline{7}$	1	0.28

Etc. up to No. 259

(Source: Sato Institute of Dental Research)

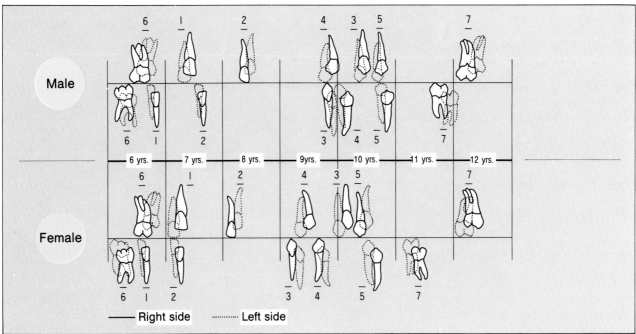

Fig. 9. Eruption Time and Eruption Order of Permanent Teeth

(Source: Kyosuke Saito)

Table 6. Eruption Order of First Molars and Incisors

	Eruption Order	N	Percentage
(1)	$\frac{}{6}\frac{6}{}\ \frac{}{1}\frac{1}{}\ \frac{}{2}\frac{2}{}$	233	65.4%
(2)	$\frac{}{6}\frac{6}{}\ \frac{}{1}\frac{}{2}\frac{1}{}\frac{2}{}$	71	19.9
(3)	$\frac{}{1}\frac{6}{6}\frac{1}{}\ \frac{}{2}\frac{2}{}$	10	2.81
(4)	$\frac{}{1}\frac{6}{6}\frac{}{2}\frac{1}{}\frac{2}{}$	9	2.25
⋮	Up to 18 eruption orders		

Table 7. Eruption Order of Canines and First and Second Premolars

	Eruption Order	N	Percentage
(1)	$\frac{}{3}\frac{}{4}\frac{4}{}\frac{3}{}\ \frac{}{5}\frac{5}{}$	26	7.30%
(2)	$\frac{}{3}\frac{4}{4}\frac{}{}\frac{3}{5}\frac{5}{}$	22	6.18
(3)	$\frac{}{3}\frac{4}{}\frac{3}{4}\ \frac{}{5}\frac{5}{}$	15	4.21
(4)	$\frac{}{3}\frac{}{4}\frac{4}{}\frac{3}{}\frac{5}{5}$	14	3.93
(5)	$\frac{}{3}\frac{4}{}\frac{3}{4}\frac{}{5}\frac{5}{}$	14	3.93
⋮	Up to 92 eruption orders		

Table 8. Eruption Order of Second Premolars and Second Molars

	Eruption Order	N	Percentage
(1)	$\frac{}{5}\frac{5}{}\ \frac{}{7}\frac{7}{}$	26	32.87%
(2)	$\frac{5}{}\frac{}{5}\frac{}{7}\frac{7}{}$	22	17.42
(3)	$\frac{}{7}\frac{}{5}\frac{5}{}\frac{7}{}$	15	3.65
(4)	$\frac{}{5}\frac{}{7}\frac{5}{}\frac{7}{}$	14	8.15
(5)	$\frac{5}{}\frac{}{5}\frac{7}{}\frac{}{7}$	14	10.39

Part II   ERUPTION OF INDIVIDUAL PERMANENT TEETH

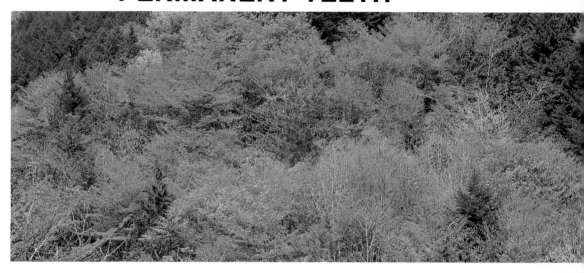

1 MAXILLARY FIRST MOLARS

Maxillary First Molars

The average eruption time for maxillary first molars is approximately 4 to 8 years of age, and these erupt on the distal side of the primary maxillary second molars. The maxillary first molar has the widest occlusal surface of all the maxillary permanent teeth and two cusps on both the buccal and lingual surfaces. The eruption order of the cusps is: mesiobuccal cusp; mesiolingual cusp; distobuccal cusp; and, finally, the distolingual cusp. The transition from gingival emergence to full eruption of the occlusal surface requires about 30 to 32 weeks (7.5 months) and sometimes as long as 12 months.

Notes on Anatomical Form and Occlusal Surfaces

1. The crowns have rounded corners and are shaped like parallel squares or diamonds.
2. There are four cusps: the mesiobuccal and distobuccal cusps on the buccal side, and the mesiolingual and distolingual cusps on the lingual side.

3. With regard to occlusion, the occlusal surface consists of a central sulcus, distal small sulci, two buccal cusps, and two lingual cusps which run along triangular ridges.
4. The central sulcus, small sulci, and fissures are deeper than those found in the premolars and form a more complex occlusal surface.

ERUPTION OF RIGHT MAXILLARY FIRST MOLAR
(Girl, age 5 years, 11 months at start of eruption)

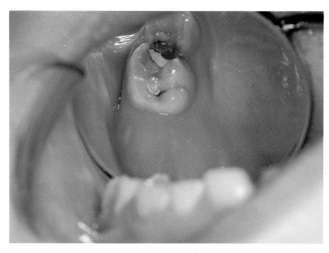

Fig. 1. The gingiva on the distal side of the primary second molar swells just prior to eruption of the first molar, which can be seen beginning at the mesiobuccal cusp.

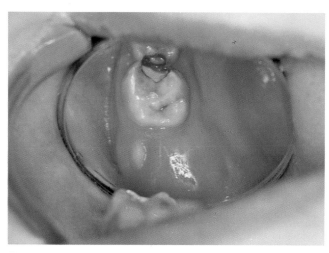

Fig. 2. 3 weeks later: the gingiva near the mesiolingual cusp swells.

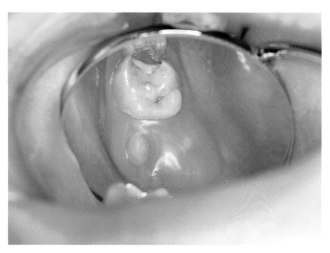

Fig. 3. 4 weeks later: the mesiobuccal cusp gradually erupts and gingiva near the erupting mesiolingual cusp swells.

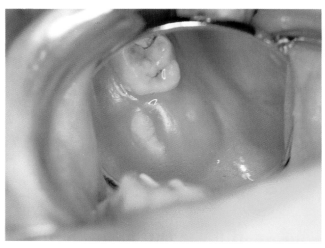

Fig. 4. 5 weeks (about 1 month) later: eruption has progressed from the mesiobuccal cusp to part of the buccal cusp and the beginnings of mesiolingual cusp eruption is visible on the gingiva surface, which appears anemic under the pressure of the erupting cusp.

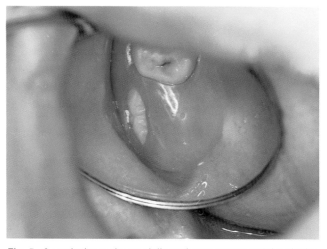

Fig. 5. 6 weeks later: the mesiolingual cusp erupts and the gingiva shows blood congestion.

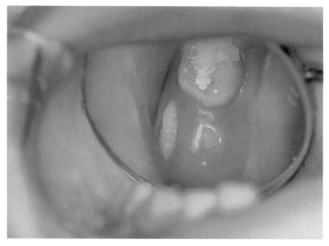

Fig. 6. 7 weeks later: the buccal cusps erupt further, and eruption of the mesiolingual cusp is more conspicuous.

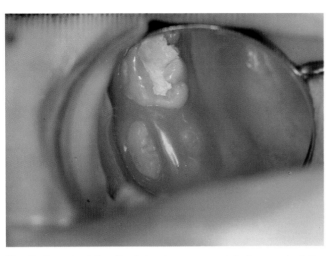

Fig. 7. 8 weeks later: the buccal cusps erupt further; part of the occlusal surface is visible.

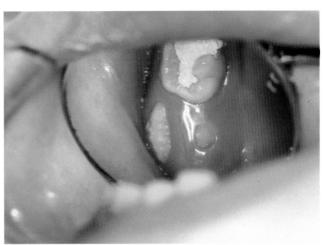

Fig. 8. 9 weeks (about 2 months) later: the buccal cusps and mesiolingual cusp erupt further and the very swollen gingiva, in center, crosses from mesial to distal sides.

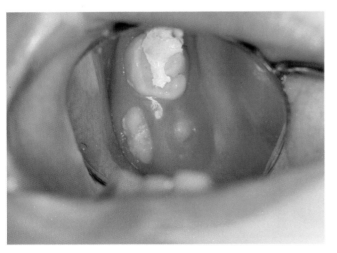

Fig. 9. 10 weeks later: part of the occlusal surface becomes visible as lingual cusps erupt further.

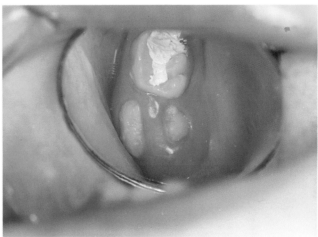

Fig. 10. 11 weeks later: rapid eruption of the occlusal surface gradually reduces the gingiva in the center.

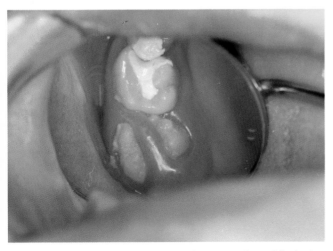

Fig. 11. 12 weeks (about 3 months) later: eruption of both the buccal and lingual cusps is nearly complete and there is further contraction of gingiva in center.

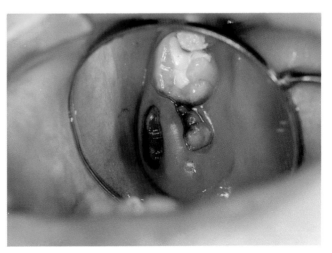

Fig. 12. 12 weeks later: the tooth is dyed with safranine and the stain is concentrated on the occlusal surface around gingiva in center. (The occlusal surface was still low and had not yet reached the occlusal line — this makes disinfection and cleaning difficult during this period.)

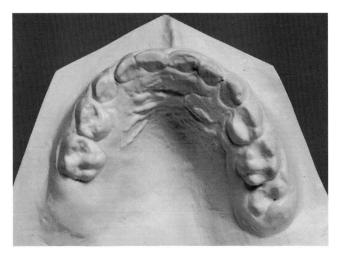

Fig. 13. At 5 years, 4 months: the left first molar erupts beginning at the mesial cusp. (Study No. 199; bimonthly mold series).

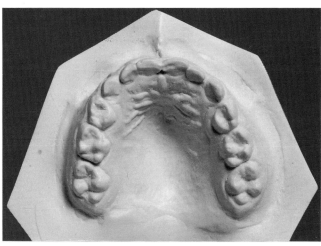

Fig. 14. At 5 years, 6 months: 2 months later, most of the occlusal surface erupts rapidly (No. 199).

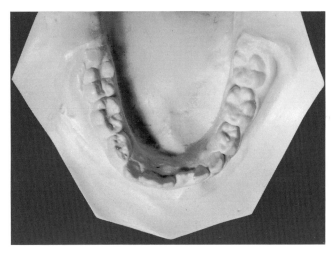

Fig. 15. At 5 years, 6 months: the mandibular central incisors are also erupting (No. 199).

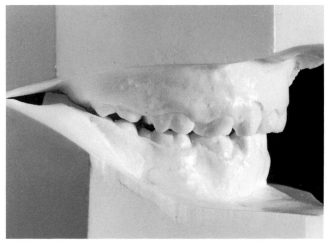

Fig. 16. At 5 years, 6 months: neither the maxillary nor the mandibular first molars have reached the occlusal line (No. 199).

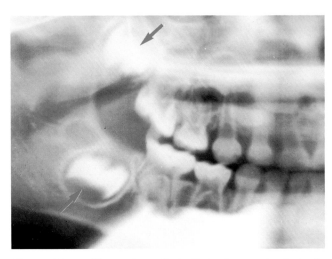

Fig. 17. The maxillary and mandibular first molars are developing in opposite directions: the maxillary first molar is forming distally and the mandibular first molar is forming mesially (2 years, 11 months).

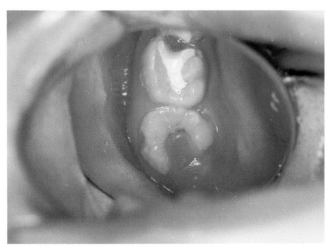

Fig. 18. 13 weeks (about 3 months) later: the gingiva breaks on the mesial side and contracts toward the distal side, as the occlusal surface erupts from the distal side to the center. Notice the poor oral hygiene that persists in this area between week 13 and 20.

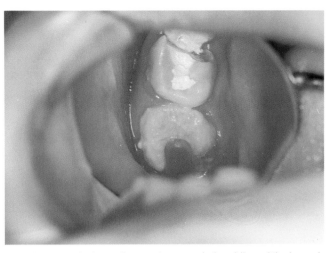

Fig. 19. 14 weeks later: the gum has receded rapidly and the buccal and lingual cusps have almost fully erupted. At the same time, about 80% of the occlusal surface, from the central sulcus to the distal groove, has erupted.

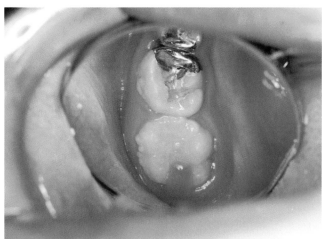

Fig. 20. 15 weeks later: the gingiva has receded almost completely, but still blocks the distal groove.

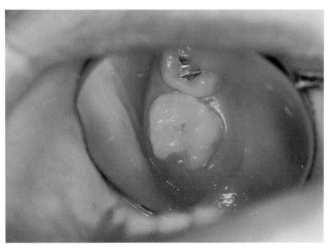

Fig. 21. 16 weeks later: little change has taken place.

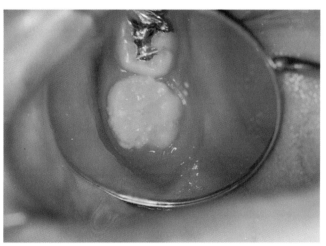

Fig. 22. 17 weeks (about 4 months) later: the occlusal surface is almost completely exposed, except for the distal marginal ridge.

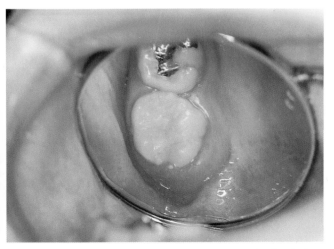

Fig. 23. 19 weeks later: some gingiva still remains at the distal edge.

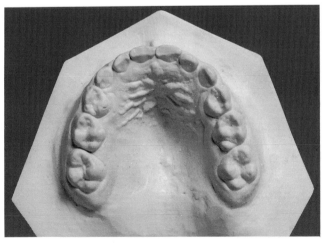

Fig. 24. At 6 years, 8 months: the occlusal surface of the first molar has erupted almost completely (No. 199).

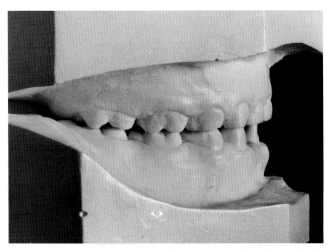

Fig. 25. At 6 years, 8 months: the primary molars have finally reached the occlusal plane, but the relation betweeen tooth 1 and 2 (Class I Angle) is still not established (No. 199).

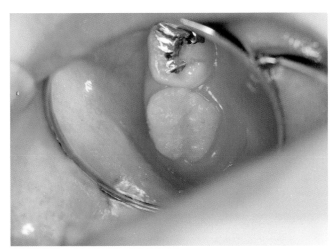

Fig. 26. 20 weeks later: the distal edge has still not erupted completely.

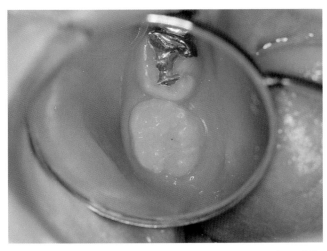

Fig. 27. 24 weeks later: the occlusal surface appears to have fully erupted; however, some gingiva still remains at the distal edge.

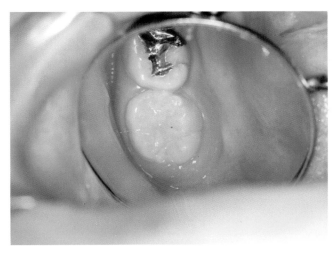

Fig. 28. 25 weeks (about 6 months) later: the distal edge of the occlusal surface has still not erupted completely.

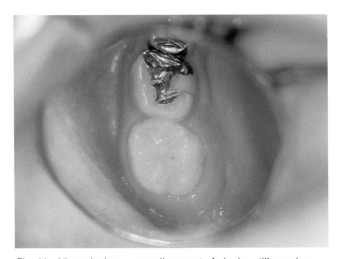

Fig. 29. 27 weeks later: a small amount of gingiva still remains.

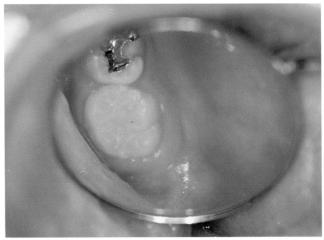

Fig. 30. 28 weeks (about 6.5 months) later: the gingiva appears to be receding from the distal edge.

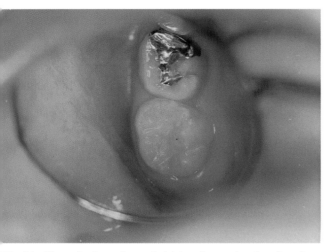

Fig. 31. 32 weeks (over 7 months) later: the occlusal surface has fully erupted — this demonstrates the long period required for eruption of the maxillary first molar's occlusal surface.

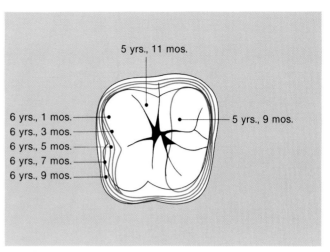

Fig. 32. Eruption process of the maxillary first molar's occlusal surface (typical diagram).

5 yrs., 11 mos.

6 yrs., 1 mos.
6 yrs., 3 mos.
6 yrs., 5 mos.
6 yrs., 7 mos.
6 yrs., 9 mos.

5 yrs., 9 mos.

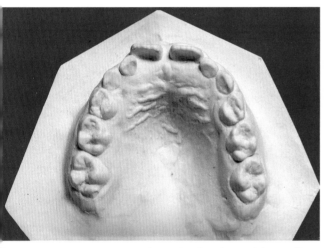

Fig. 33. At 6 years, 8 months: the occlusal surfaces of the maxillary first permanent molars have erupted completely.

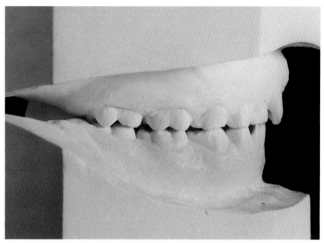

Fig. 34. At 6 years, 8 months: the maxillary and mandibular first molars are not fully occluded.

Clinical Memo

1. Just prior to eruption of the first molar, the gingiva on the distal side of the second primary molar swells up considerably.
2. Eruption stage 1: the tooth erupts from the mesiobuccal cusp to the buccal cusp (1 to 5 weeks after initial swelling).
3. Eruption stage 2: part of the mesiolingual cusp erupts. The gingiva forms a wide bridge that covers the tooth's central groove and distolingual cusp (6 to 11 weeks).
4. Eruption stage 3: the central gingiva bridge is broken, and about two-thirds of the occlusal surface has emerged. During this stage, the gingiva is easily contaminated and most difficult to clean, which raises the risk of caries (12 to 15 weeks).
5. Eruption stage 4: the occlusal surface is at least two-thirds erupted and only the distal edge remains covered. It is during this stage that caries prevention is most important, using such methods as fluoride treatment, fissure sealants, preventive fillings, and dental hygiene counseling — all of which are likely to prove effective (15th to 20th week of eruption).
6. Eruption stage 5: the occlusal surface erupts completely, including the distal edge, but the tooth does not yet arrive at the occlusal plane with the opposite molar and, thus, is susceptible to accumulation of food particles. It is also difficult to clean this tooth with an ordinary toothbrush; hence, a molar brush is recommended (21 to 28 weeks).

2 MANDIBULAR FIRST MOLARS

Mandibular First Molars

The average eruption time for the mandibular first molars is approximately 4 to 8 years of age. These molars are the first of the permanent teeth to erupt. Eruption begins from the mesiobuccal cusp and occurs behind the primary second molar.

Their occlusal surfaces are the largest among the permanent teeth and consist of five cusps which are listed here in order of their eruption: the mesiobuccal cusp; the mesiolingual cusp; the distobuccal cusp; the distolingual cusp; and the distal cusp. The transition from gingival emergence to full eruption of the occlusal surface takes about 12 months, and sometimes longer, making these molars the slowest to erupt of the permanent teeth.

Notes on Anatomical Form and Occlusal Surfaces

1. The crowns have rounded corners and are shaped like parallel squares or diamonds.
2. There are five cusps; the mesiobuccal and distobuccal + distal cusps, on the buccal side, and the mesiolingual and distolingual cusps, on the lingual side.
3. With regard to occlusion, the occlusal surface consists of a central sulcus, mesial and distal small sulci, these buccal cusps and two lingual cusps which run along triangular ridges.
4. The central sulcus, small sulci, and fissures are deeper than those found in the molars and form a more complex occlusal surface.

ERUPTION OF LEFT MANDIBULAR FIRST MOLAR
(Girl, age 5 years, 4 months at start of eruption)

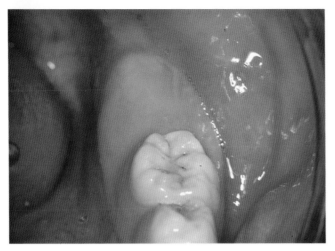

Fig. 1. The mandibular first molar begins to erupt on the distal side of the primary second molar, and prior to eruption, the gingiva swells and the area appears anemic.

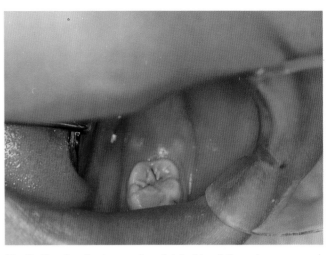

Fig. 2. Eruption begins on the distal side of the primary second molar as the first molar's mesiobuccal and mesiolingual cusps begin to emerge.

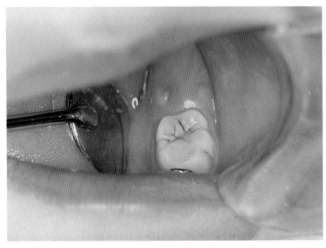

Fig. 3. 1 week later: the mesiobuccal and mesiolingual cusps have emerged only slightly.

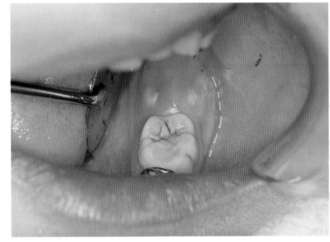

Fig. 4. 2 weeks later: the two mesial cusps gradually emerge.

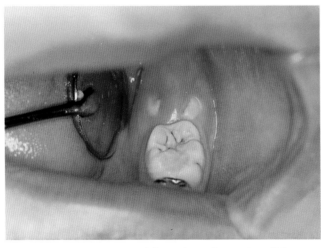

Fig. 5. 3 weeks later: the mesiobuccal cusp is erupting a little more rapidly than the mesiolingual cusp.

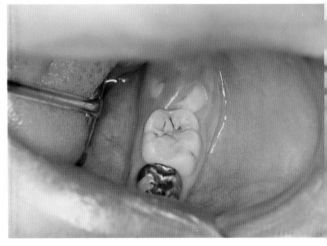

Fig. 6. 4 weeks (about 1 month) later: eruption has reached the mesial edge, and the gingiva in this area has become swollen.

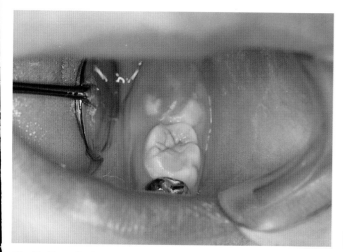

Fig. 7. 5 weeks later: the mesiobuccal cusp has fully erupted and the gingiva has receded to where only a small amount still remains on the mesial edge.

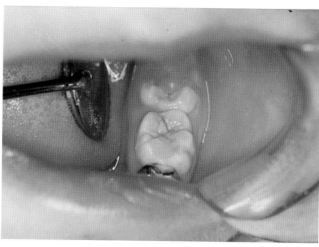

Fig. 8. 6 weeks (about 1.5 months) later: the gingiva has broken away from the mesial edge and is receding quickly. The mesial cusps have further erupted and part of the mesial groove and mesial sulcus can be seen.

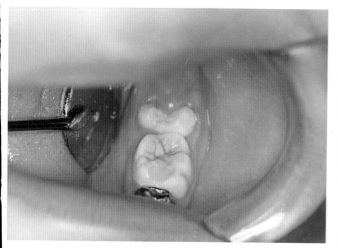

Fig. 9. 7 weeks later: eruption of the mesial cusps and the occlusal surface progresses further.

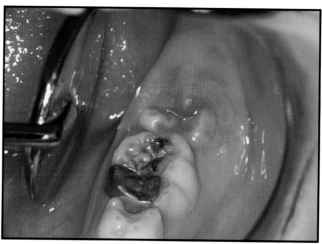

Fig. 10. 6 weeks later: colored with fuchsine dye, the stain is concentrated from the gingival edge to the mesial groove area (Patient No. 205).

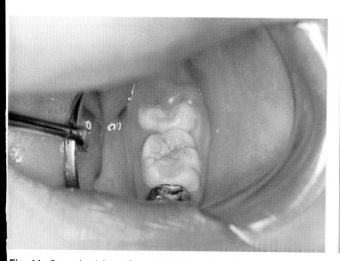

Fig. 11. 8 weeks (about 2 months) later: the gingiva has receded further and eruption reaches toward the distobuccal cusp and the central sulcus.

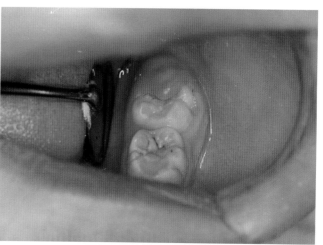

Fig. 12. 9 weeks later: the mesiobuccal cusp as fully emerged and part of the distobuccal cusp is visible. The mesiobuccal groove and central sulcus can also be seen.

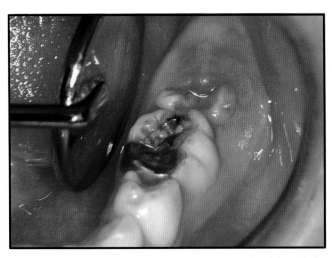

Fig. 13. During the 9th week, fuchsine dye is applied and the stain is concentrated from the gingival edge to the central sulcus and central grooves (Patent No. 205).

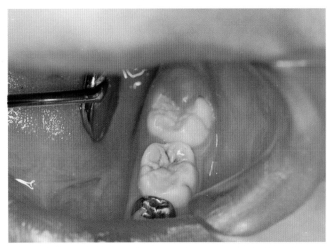

Fig. 14. 10 weeks (about 2 months) later: part of the distolingual cusp can be seen and about four-fifths of the occlusal surface has erupted.

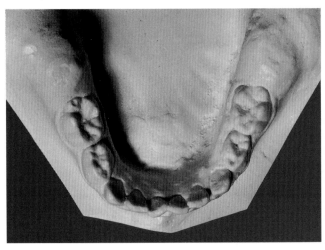

Fig. 15. At 5 years, 2 months: the gingiva is swollen prior to eruption of the first molars (No. 199).

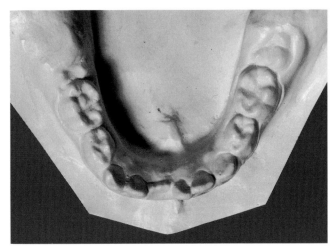

Fig. 16. At 5 years, 4 months: 2 months later, the mesiobuccal and mesiolingual cusps have already emerged (No. 199).

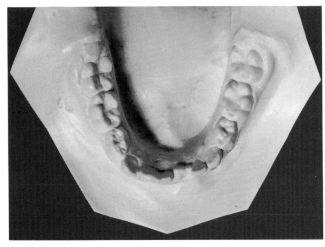

Fig. 17. At 5 years, 6 months: 2 months later, the mesiolingual cusps and all four buccal cusps have emerged, although gingiva still covers the distal sulcus.

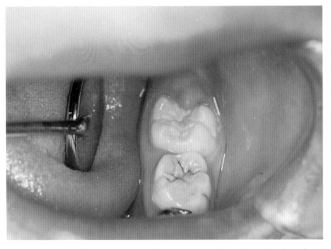

Fig. 18. 12 weeks later: the gingiva over the distal edge has receded further (No. 199).

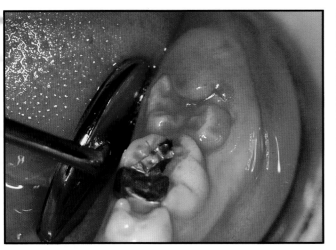

Fig. 19. During the 12th week, fuchsine dye is applied and the stain is concentrated on the gingival edge and the central sulcus (Patient No. 205).

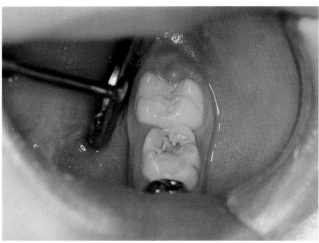

Fig. 20. 13 weeks (about 3 months) later: eruption has progressed to the distobuccal and distolingual cusps and to part of the distal edge.

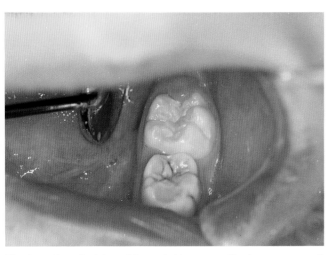

Fig. 21. 15 weeks (about 3.5 months) later: eruption has progressed at the distobuccal cusp and most of the occlusal surface has erupted.

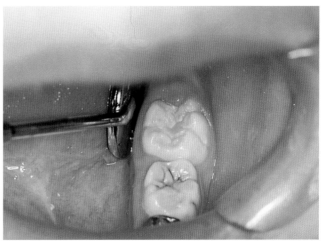

Fig. 22. 16 weeks later: some gingiva remains on the distal edge.

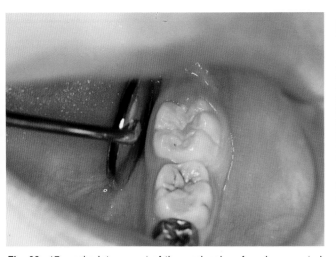

Fig. 23. 17 weeks later: most of the occlusal surface has erupted and eruption has progressed to the distal groove.

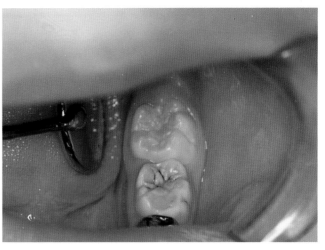

Fig. 24. 18 weeks later: still some gingiva remains on the distal edge.

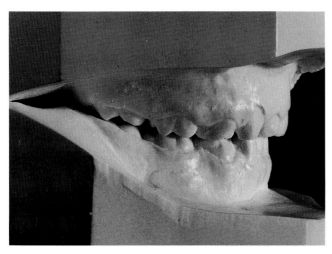

Fig. 25. At 5 years, 6 months: one-to-one opposite relation is shown between the maxillary and mandibular first molars, although they are not yet fully occluded (No. 199).

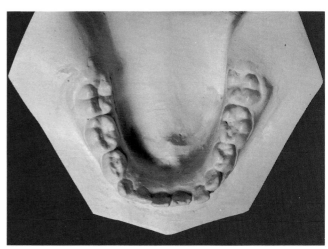

Fig. 26. At 6 years: 8 months after the beginning of eruption, the distal edge has still not erupted completely (No. 199).

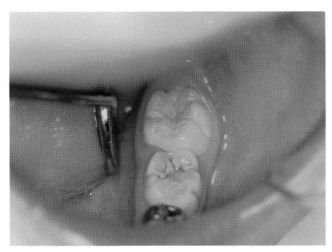

Fig. 27. 20 weeks later: some gingiva still remains on the distal edge.

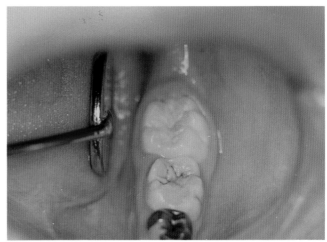

Fig. 28. 21 weeks later: the distal edge can finally be seen and the occlusal surface has almost completely erupted; however, some gingiva still remains on the distal edge.

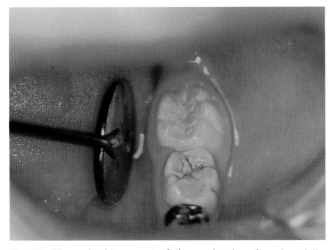

Fig. 29. 22 weeks later: most of the occlusal surface has fully erupted.

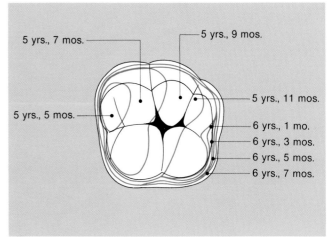

Fig. 30. Eruption process of the mandibular first molar's occlusal surface (Typical diagram).

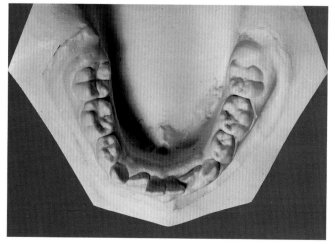 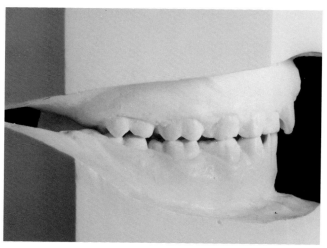

Fig. 31. At 6 years, 2 months: eruption is still not complete — even after 10 months (No. 199).

Fig. 32. At 6 years, 8 months: the occlusal line has been reached, but the teeth are meeting in a one-to-one opposite relationship instead of interdigitating (No. 199).

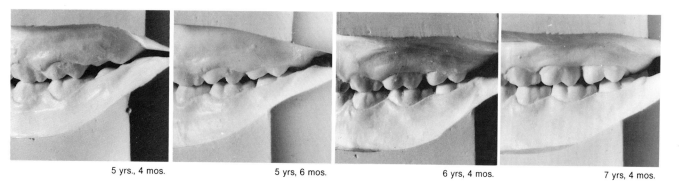

| 5 yrs., 4 mos. | 5 yrs, 6 mos. | 6 yrs, 4 mos. | 7 yrs, 4 mos. |

Fig. 33. Phases of occlusion of the maxillary and mandibular first molars (No. 199).

Figs. 10, 13 and 19 are not of the same patient with that of the other illustrations.

Eruption of First Molars

The first molars are the earliest to erupt of the permanent teeth, and they appear on the distal side of the primary second molars. Because they erupt into relatively normal positions, they are said to be the key to the formation of permanent occlusion.

1. Eruption of the maxillary and mandibular first molars occurs early, between the ages of 4 and 8. (See Table 1; pp. 2, 26, and 27; and Figs. 34 and 35.)
2. The period between the start and completion of eruption is a long one, ranging from 5 months to as long as 36 months (3 years). The average eruption period is 11 months for maxillary first molars and 17 months for mandibular first molars. (See Table 1; Figs. 32 and 33; and p. 42.)
3. The eruption direction of the maxillary first molars is buccal and that of the mandibular first molars is mesiolingual. These first molars gradually move next to the distal surface of the primary second molars and toward the occlusal surface of the primary molars.
4. The first molars take a long time to occlude: from 2 to 3 years, including the time required for eruption of the occlusal surfaces.
5. During eruption, the first molars have a low occlusal level and temporarily do not occlude when the occluding teeth have not yet erupted.
6. During eruption, part of the occlusal surface is covered by gingiva which makes the teeth prone to contamination.

Relation Between First Molars and Primary Second Molars

Although all of the first molars erupt toward the distal surface of the primary second molars, the maxillary and mandibular first molars differ in the way they are formed and in the way they emerge from their respective bony crypts.

1. The maxillary first molars are distally oriented during their formation and eruption toward the primary second molars. After their eruption has begun, they move downward, approximating the distal surface of the primary second molars, and gradually rotate mesially as they reach the primary occlusal line (see Fig. 36 on p. 28).

   The mandibular first molars are mesially oriented during their formation and eruption, and remain so, until they reach the primary occlusal line (see Fig. 37 on p. 28).
2. Relation between terminal plane and first molars: There is a relation between the distal surfaces of the maxillary and mandibular primary second molars at the time of occlusion and the eruption time of first molars. When the mandibular primary second molars' distal surfaces interdigitate mesially with their maxillary counterparts, this is called a mesial step type. If the two meet on the same plane, it is called the vertical type, and if the mandibular primary second molars interdigitate distally, it is called the distal step type.

   In the case of the mesial step type, when the first molars erupt, they usually occlude normally, as long as the mesial step is not too extreme. Primary molar occlusion is also usually normal in the case of the vertical step type. However, the distal step type often leads to a Class II malocclusion.

   Therefore, in cases where four or five-year-olds have decayed or missing primary teeth, resulting in abnormal occlusion, this invites the first molars to drift mesially and does not leave sufficient leeway for the eruption of laterally erupting teeth, which in turn can cause malocclusion. Even after the first molars have finished erupting, premature loss of a primary first or second molar can easily lead to mesial drifting which must be controlled not only in patients of ages 4 to 6 but in all those for whom laterally erupting teeth have not yet finished erupting.

Table 1. First Molar Eruption Times

			Age 4.0~ 4.11	5.0~ 5.11	6.0~ 6.11	7.0~ 7.11	8.0~ 8.11
Maxillary	Male	98	0.0%	13.3%	54.1%	29.6%	3.1%
	Female	112	0.9	16.1	58.0	23.2	1.8
	Total	210	0.5	14.8	56.2	26.2	2.4
Mandibular	Male	98	2.0%	24.5%	53.1%	17.3%	3.1%
	Female	112	1.8	37.5	50.9	8.9	1.9
	Total	210	1.9	31.4	51.9	12.9	1.9

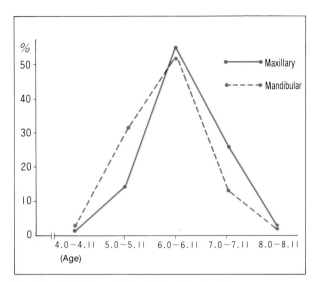

Fig. 34. Distribution of First Molar Eruption Times.
(Source: Sato Institute of Dental Research)

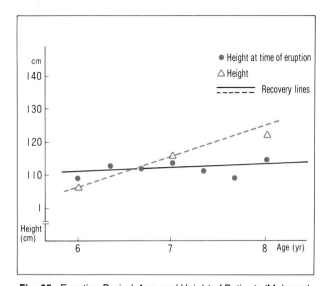

Fig. 35. Eruption Period, Age, and Height of Patients (Male and Female) with Erupting Maxillary First Molars.
(Source: Inoue)

Table 2. Relation between Maxillary First Molar Eruption Time and Height.

Age at Start of Eruption	Height (cm)	Age at Start of Eruption	Height (cm)
6.0~6.3 Age	108.9 cm	7.0~7.2 Age	113.6 cm
6.4~6.7	112.3	7.4~7.7	110.2
6.8~6.11	112.3	7.8~7.11	109.1
		8.0~8.3	113.1

(Source: Inoue)

Table 3. Relation of Distal Surfaces in Maxillary and Mandibular Primary Second Molars

		Source: Sato 196 cases	Source: Yamashita et al.
Both sides	V	53.57	59.1
Both sides	M	17.34	19.1
Both sides	D	0.51	4.6
One side	V		
One side	M	26.02	9.1
One side	V		
One side	M	22.55	8.1
		(1951)	(1960)

V : Vertical type

M: Mesial type

D : Distal type

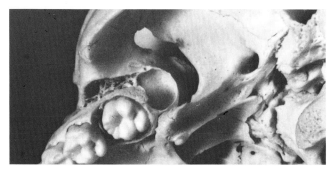
Fig. 36. Distally Oriented Eruption of Maxillary First Molar Crown

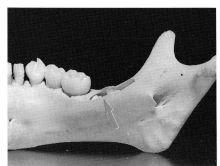

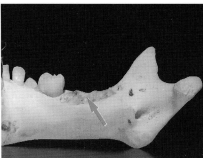

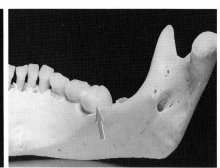

A. Crown begins to erupt from the alveolus.

B. Occlusal surface is lingually oriented at start of eruption.

C. After eruption, the first molar is mesially oriented in line with the row of primary teeth.

Fig. 37. Eruption Orientations of Mandibular First Molar Crowns

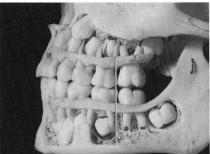

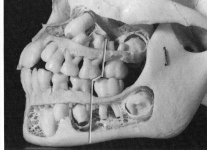

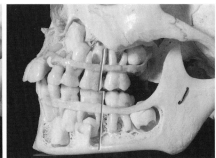

A. Vertical type

B. Mesial type

C. Distal type

Fig. 38. Relation of Distal Surfaces of Maxillary and Mandibular Primary Second Molars

Clinical Memo

1. Just prior to the mandibular molar's eruption, the gingiva on the distal side of the primary second molar becomes swollen.
2. Eruption stage 1: The mesiobuccal and lingual cusps are slightly erupted, and local gingival swelling indicates the difficulty of occlusion with the gingiva present (1 to 3 weeks after initial eruption).
3. Eruption stage 2: The mesiobuccal and lingual cusps have erupted form the mesial edge to the mesial sulcus. Cleaning the crown is difficult during this stage, and the crown is easily contaminated by accumulated food particles (4 to 7 weeks).
4. Eruption stage 3: Eruption has progressed to the occlusal surface's central sulcus. The gingiva still covers the crown's edges, which makes them extremely conducive to decay and difficult to clean. Caries occur quite easily during this stage, and, thus, utmost caution should be taken (8 to 10 weeks).
5. Eruption stage 4: Eruption has progressed to at least two-thirds of the occlusal surface, or, up to the distal edge. Since the crown's sulci and grooves are exposed, cleaning is now possible. Therefore, during this stage, dental hygiene counseling should be practiced, along with fluoride treatments, and other treatment as needed (11 to 20 weeks).
6. Eruption stage 5: Although the occlusal surfaces have fully erupted, maxillary and mandibular occlusion has still not been reached; and therefore, patients should be advised of the need to brush carefully the occlusal surfaces.

3 MAXILLARY SECOND MOLARS

Maxillary Second Molars

The average eruption time for maxillary second molars is approximately 11 years of age. As eruption occurs, the buccal cusp will emerge. There are four cusps at the occlusal surface. In order of eruption, they are the mesiobuccal cusp, the mesiolingual cusp, the distobuccal cusp, and finally, the lingual cusp. The transition from gingival emergence to full eruption of the occlusal surface takes 20 to 25 weeks (5 to 7 months), which is much faster than the eruption of the maxillary first molar.

Notes on Anatomical Form and Occlusal Surfaces

1. The crown's edges are very dull and the entire crown has a nearly round appearance.
2. The cusps are small and low.
3. The distobuccal and distolingual cusps are especially prone to degeneration. In some cases, these cusps fail to appear, leaving only three cusps in the crown. Accordingly, there are many cases in which maxillary second molars appear, but with abnormal anatomical forms.

ERUPTION OF RIGHT MAXILLARY SECOND MOLAR
(Girl, age 11 years, 10 months, at start of eruption)

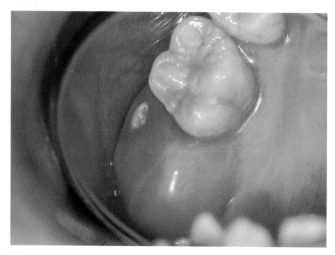

Fig. 1. Eruption, on the distal side of the first molar, begins with the emergence of the mesiobuccal cusp.

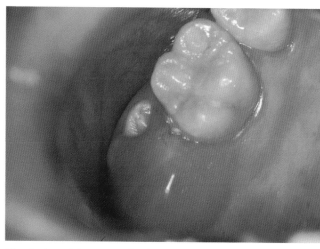

Fig. 2. 1 week later: eruption has progressed to include a triangular groove that is part of the occlusal surface.

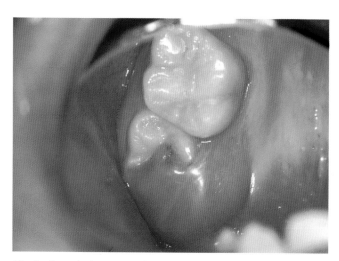

Fig. 3. 2 weeks later: eruption progresses quickly. The gingiva has receded across part of the occlusal surface; the distobuccal cusp and part of the mesiolingual cusp emerged.

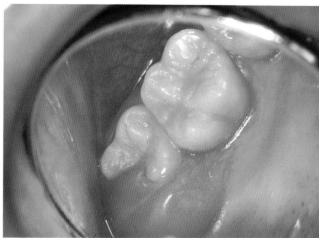

Fig. 4. 3 weeks later: most of the distobuccal cusp and about two-thirds of the mesiolingual cusp have emerged, along with the central sulcus of the occlusal surface.

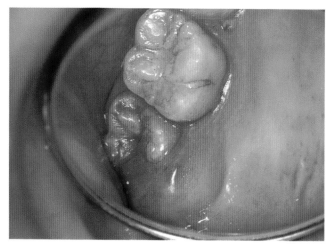

Fig. 5. About 3 weeks later: fuchsine dye shows stains at the gingival edge and in the central sulcus of the occlusal surface.

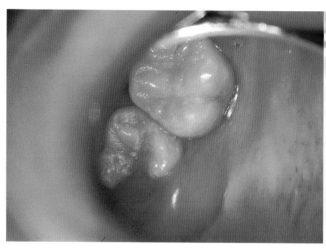

Fig. 6. 4 weeks (about 1 month) later: the gingiva has receded further, exposing almost all of the mesiolingual cusp.

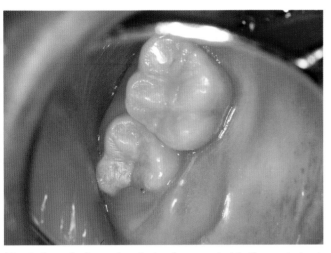

Fig. 7. 5 weeks later: the gingiva has receded further and about four-fifths of the occlusal surface is now exposed.

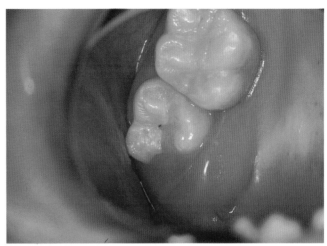

Fig. 8. 7 weeks later: the occlusal surface has erupted further.

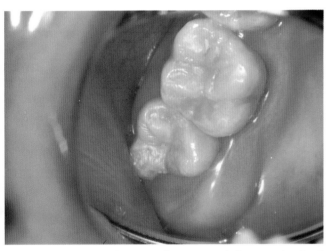

Fig. 9. 8 weeks later: the crown has emerged almost to the distal edge.

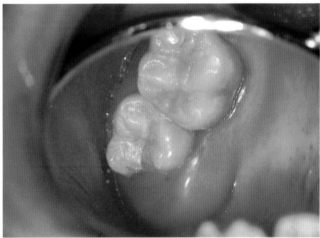

Fig. 10. 9 weeks (2 months) later: the distal edge has still not fully emerged.

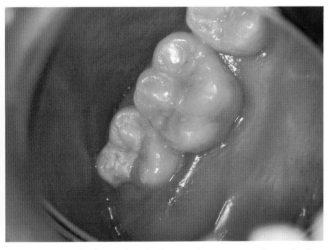

Fig. 11. 10 weeks later: the gingiva continues to recede gradually.

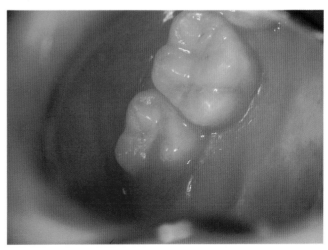

Fig. 12. 11 weeks later: almost all of the occlusal surface has emerged, although the distolingual cusp remains covered.

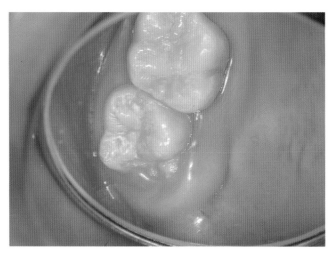

Fig. 13. 13 weeks (3 months) later: the distal edge is still partially covered by gingiva and the occlusal surface is still not fully erupted.

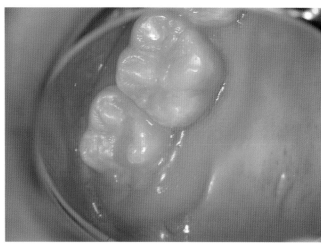

Fig. 14. 13 weeks (3 months) later: the distal edge is still partially covered by gingiva and the occlusal surface is still not fully erupted.

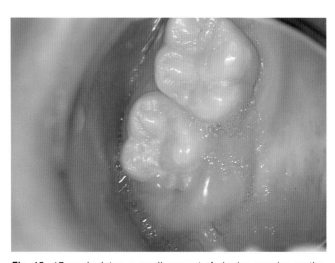

Fig. 15. 17 weeks later: a small amount of gingiva remains on the distal edge.

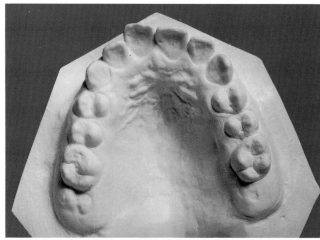

Fig. 16. At 10 years, 8 months: the right maxillary second molar begins erupting with the emergence of the mesiobuccal cusp (No. 199).

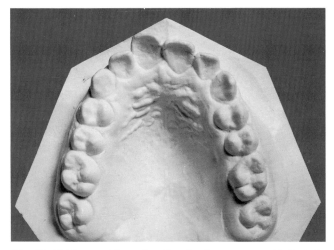

Fig. 17. At 10 years, 10 months: Eruption has progressed to include the mesio — and distobuccal cusps, the mesiolingual cusp, and most of the occlusal surface. The distolingual cusps, however, remain covered. (No. 199)

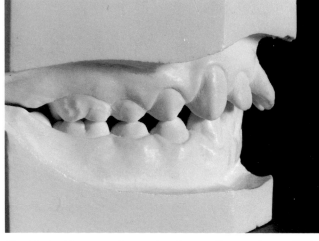

Fig. 18. At 10 years, 10 months: the maxillary and mandibular second molars are not occluding at all.

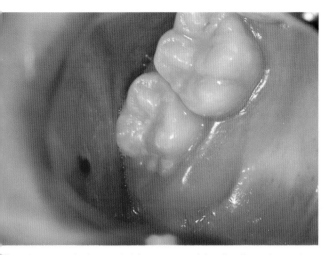

Fig. 19. 18 weeks (4 months) later: most of the distolingual cusp has emerged, but a little gingiva remains on the distal edge.

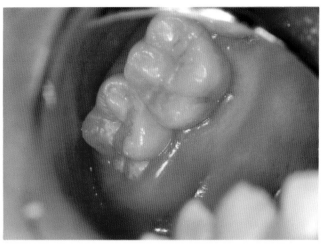

Fig. 20. 19 weeks later: virtually all of the occlusal surface has erupted, although a small amount of gingiva remains on the crown.

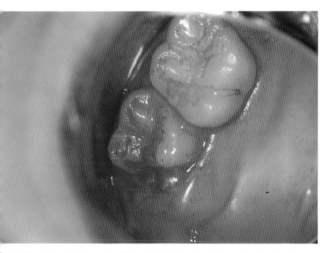

Fig. 21. About 18 weeks later: fuchsine dye is applied and shows stains in the small distal sulcus and distal grooves.

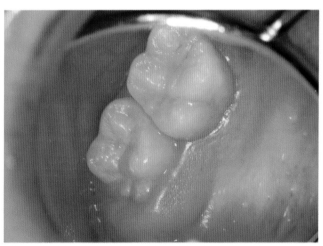

Fig. 22. 20 weeks (about 4.5 months) later: only a little gingiva remains on the crown.

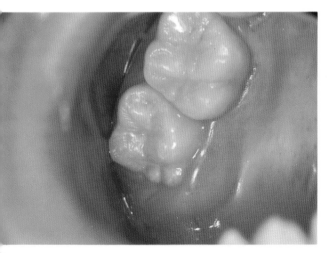

Fig. 23. 22 weeks later: almost all of the occlusal surface has erupted, and only a little gingiva remains on the crown's distal edge.

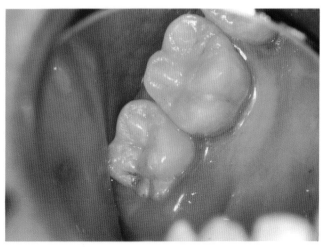

Fig. 24. 24 weeks later: the crown seems to have emerged completely, but in fact still has a little further to go. In spite of the time involved, the illustrations show very little apparent change in the process.

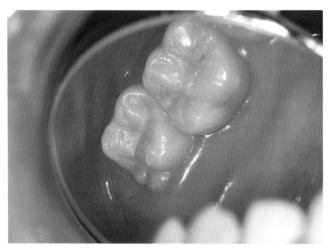

Fig. 25. 27 weeks (6 months) later: the occlusal surface has erupted completely.

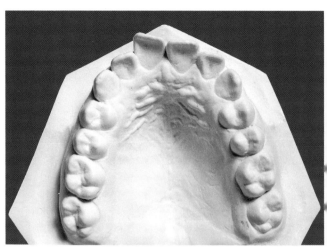

Fig. 26. At 11 years, 4 months: 8 months after initial eruption, the occlusal surface has finally erupted fully (No. 199).

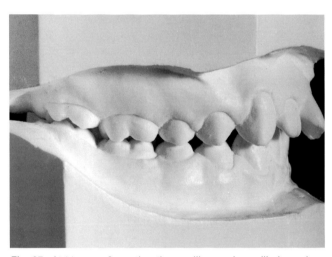

Fig. 27. At 11 years, 2 months: the maxillary and mandibular molars have still not occluded (No. 199).

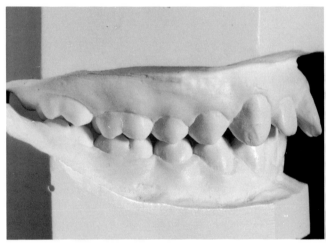

Fig. 28. 12 years, 10 months: the maxillary and mandibular second molars have occluded completely — 26 months after the start of eruption (No. 199).

Clinical Memo

1. Eruption stages 1 and 2: once their eruption has begun, the occlusal surfaces of the maxillary and mandibular second molars erupt relatively quickly. Eruption progresses from the mesiobuccal cusp to part of the distobuccal and mesiolingual cusps, and then to the occlusal surface's central sulcus and part of the central grooves. Extra care should be taken in cleaning these areas, since the occlusal surface erupts toward the distal edge of the first molars (first 3 weeks of eruption).

2. Eruption stage 3: about two-thirds of the occlusal surface has erupted, although gingiva still covers the distal edge. During this stage, thorough cleaning, combined with either preventive fillings or fluorine treatment, is recommended as a method of effective caries prevention (4th and 5th week of eruption).

3. Eruption stage 4: most of the occlusal surface has erupted while only a little gingiva still remains on the distal edge. In view of the patient's age (about 10), dental hygiene advice should be given to help prevent caries.

4. Eruption stage 5: by now, the occlusal surface should be fully erupted, although the maxillary and mandibular second molars are not yet fully occluded. It is, therefore, especially important that the patient be advised to brush the teeth properly.

4 MANDIBULAR SECOND MOLARS

Mandibular Second Molars

The average eruption time for mandibular second molars is approximately 11 years of age. The eruption order of the cusps is as follows: the mesiobuccal cusp, the mesiolingual cusp, the distobuccal cusp, and finally the distolingual cusp. The anatomical forms of these molars are similar to those of the mandibular fist molars; however, there are only four cusps on each, due to degeneration of the distal cusps. The transition from gingival emergence to full eruption of the occlusal surfaces takes 20 weeks (about 5 months), almost the same as maxillary second molars.

Notes on Anatomical Form and Occlusal Surfaces
---

1. The anatomical form is often an abnormal pentagonal shape.
2. As with the maxillary second molars, the mandibular second molars are prone to degeneration.
3. The crown's corners are rounded and degeneration of the cusps can be seen.
4. The central grooves are often crossed with the buccal and lingual grooves, and there is usually a deep central sulcus, as in the first molar.

ERUPTION OF LEFT MANDIBULAR SECOND MOLAR
(Girl, age 11 years, 9 months, at start of eruption)

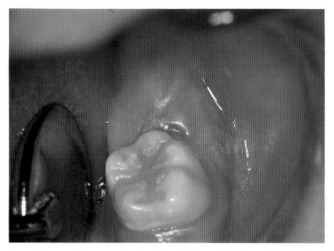

Fig. 1. Impending eruption is indicated by gingival swelling on the distal side of the first molar.

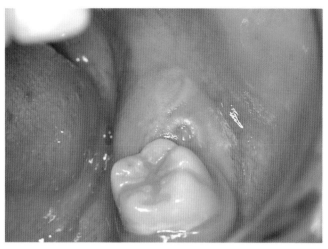

Fig. 2. Part of the mesiobuccal cusp is just barely visible. The gingiva over the occlusal surface is swollen and appears anemic.

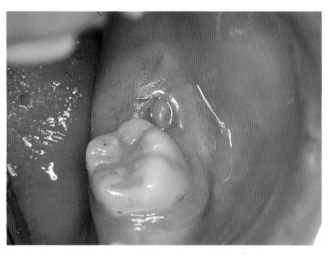

Fig. 3. 1 week later: the mesiobuccal cusp is the first to emerge.

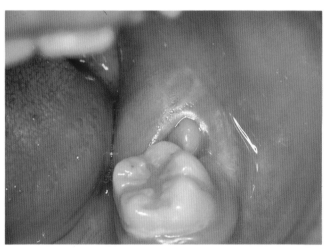

Fig. 4. 2 weeks later: the mesiobuccal cusp continues to emerge and a mesial inclination of the crown can be detected.

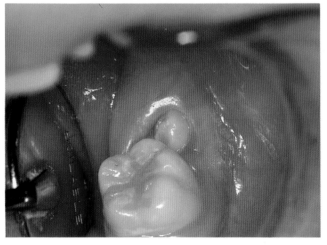

Fig. 5. 3 weeks later: the mesial edge has moved up next to the first molar's distal edge and the gingiva is receding — thereby exposing some of the occlusal surface.

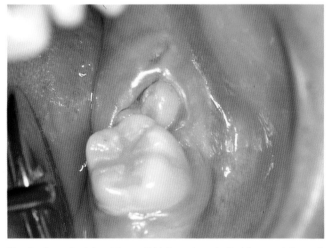

Fig. 6. 4 weeks (about 1 month) later: almost all of the mesiobuccal cusp has erupted and part of the mesiolingual cusp can be seen.

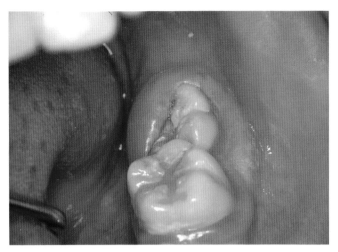

Fig. 7. 5 weeks (1 month) later: the gingiva is receding rapidly exposing about two-thirds of the distobuccal cusp and the central sulcus.

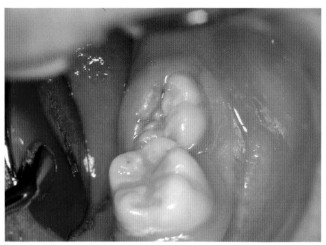

Fig. 8. 6 weeks (1.5 months): the gingiva has receded further, exposing more of the central sulcus and grooves.

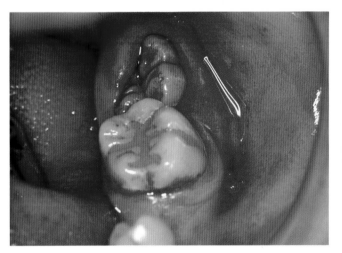

Fig. 9. During the 6th week, fuchsine dye was applied and showed the strongest stains in the central grooves and nearby smaller grooves (brushing is difficult during this period because the occlusal surface has not yet reached the occlusal line).

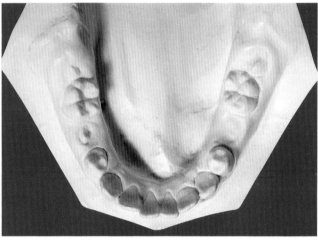

Fig. 10. At 10 years, 6 months: in the mandibular left second molar, eruption begins with the mesiobuccal cusp (No. 199).

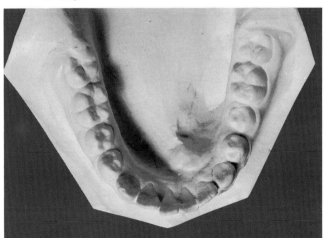

Fig. 11. At 10 years, 8 months: 2 months later, the mesiolingual and distobuccal cusps have emerged (No. 199).

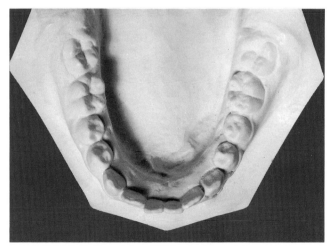

Fig. 12. At 10 years, 10 months: 2 months later, part of the occlusal surface has erupted (No. 199).

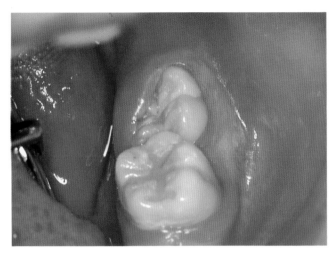

Fig. 13. 7 weeks later: the occlusal surface erupts further, exposing most of the distobuccal cusp and about three quarters of the occlusal surface.

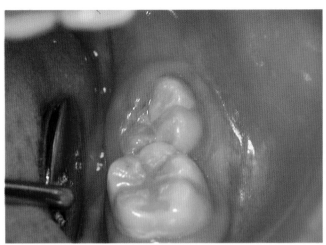

Fig. 14. 9 weeks (2 months) later: the occlusal surface is exposed from the central sulcus to the lingual groove.

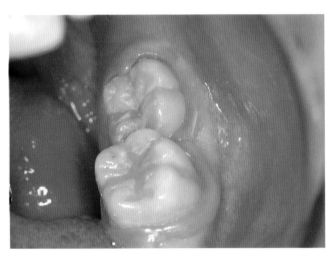

Fig. 15. 10 weeks later: eruption has progressed as far as the disto-lingual cusp, and the gingiva covers only the distal edge.

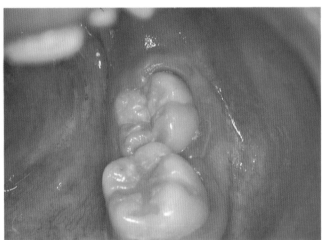

Fig. 16. 11 weeks later: only a small amount of gingiva remains on the distal edge.

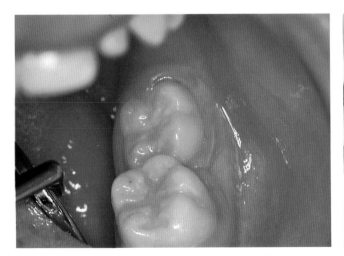

Fig. 17. 12 weeks later: much time is required for the complete eruption of the distal edge.

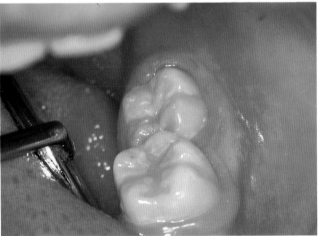

Fig. 18. 13 weeks (3 months) later: almost all of the occlusal surface has erupted, although a small amount of gingiva remains on part of the distal edge.

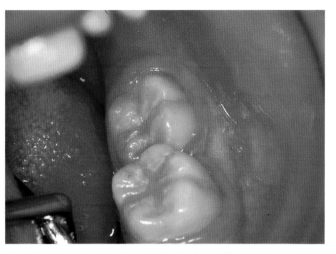

Fig. 19. 14 weeks later: the distal edge has still not fully erupted.

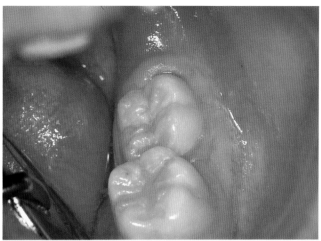

Fig. 20. 15 weeks later: some gingiva still remains on the distal edge.

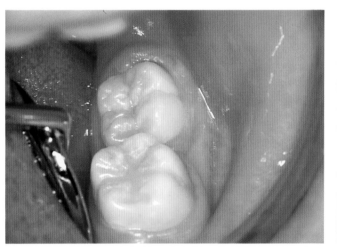

Fig. 21. 17 weeks later: there is still a bit of gingiva left on the distal edge.

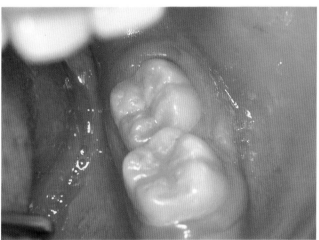

Fig. 22. 19 weeks later: nearly all of the occlusal surface has erupted.

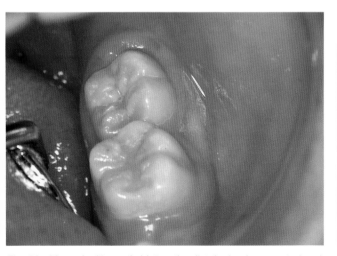

Fig. 23. 20 weeks (4 months) later: the distal edge has erupted and the occlusal surface's eruption is almost complete.

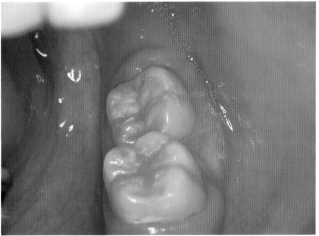

Fig. 24. 22 weeks (about 5 months) later: the remaining gingiva recedes further and the occlusal surface has completed its eruption.

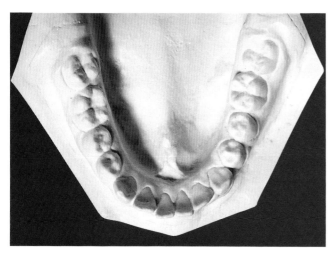

Fig. 25. At 11 years: 6 months after the initial eruption, the distolingual cusp is emerging and a small amount of gingiva covers the distal edge (No. 199).

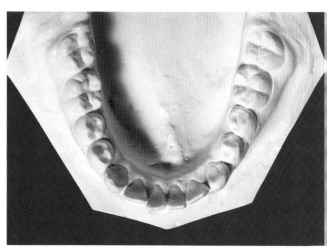

Fig. 26. At 11 years, 4 months: 10 months after the initial eruption, the occlusal surface has finally erupted completely (No. 199).

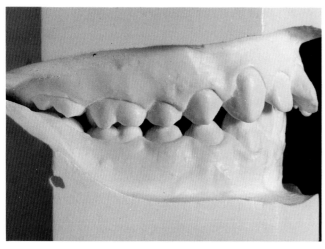

Fig. 27. At 11 years: there is not occlusion between maxillary and mandibular molars (No. 199).

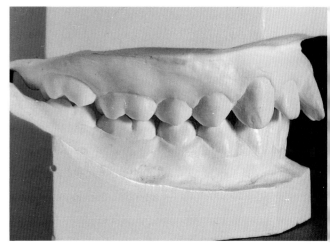

Fig. 28. At 12 years, 10 months: the maxillary and mandibular molars have occluded completely (No. 199).

Clinical Memo

1. Eruption stage 1: prior to eruption of the second molar, the gingiva on the distal side of the first molar becomes swollen. Eruption begins with the mesiobuccal cusp (first 3 weeks of eruption).
2. Eruption stage 2: a triangular area of exposed occlusal surface, accounting for about half of the total surface, has erupted. This area includes the mesial edge, the mesiolingual cusp, and the buccal cusps. At this point, the area can easily become dirty and infected (until about the 6th week of eruption).
3. Eruption stage 3: eruption has progressed relatively quickly, exposing about two-thirds of the occlusal surface. At this stage, this area easily traps food particles and is difficult to clean.
4. Eruption stages 4 and 5: most of the occlusal surface is exposed, although, in stage 4, it takes a long time for the distal edge to erupt fully (until the 22nd week of eruption).

Eruption of Second Molars

The second molars erupt on the distal side of the first molars at about the age of 11.

1. The occlusal surface eruption (from initial eruption to full eruption of the occlusal surface) of maxillary second molars takes about 8 months and that of mandibular molars about 15 months.
2. The second molars are similar to the first molars in their eruption direction; the maxillary second molars erupt with a distal inclination and the mandibular second molars with a slight mesial inclination. The occlusal surfaces of both sets of molars gradually correct their inclination and meet the first molars' occlusal plane.
3. Occlusion of the maxillary and mandibular second molars is relatively slow, requiring from one to two years after initial eruption.
4. During eruption, the second molars' occlusal surfaces are low and do not occlude.
5. During the eruption period, gingiva covers part of the occlusal surface, rendering it especially prone to infection.

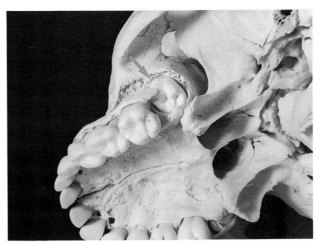

Fig. 29. Eruption Direction of Second Molars (6 years).

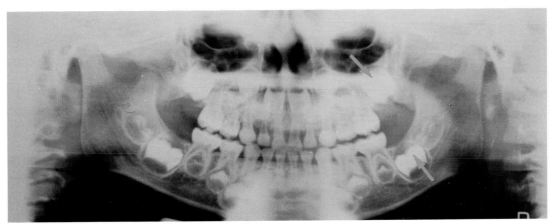

Fig. 30. Formation of Second Molars (4 years, 3 months).

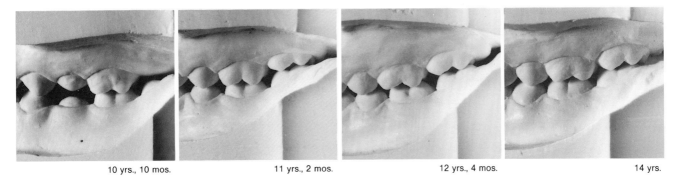

| 10 yrs., 10 mos. | 11 yrs., 2 mos. | 12 yrs., 4 mos. | 14 yrs. |

Fig. 31. Phases in the Occlusion of Second Molars.
(No. 199).

Table 1. First Molar Eruption Start Time and Occlusal Surface Eruption Completion Time.

Jaws	Period Sex	Eruption Start Time N	Average	Completion N	Average	Period N	Average
Maxillary	Male	43	6. 6 yrs.	37	7.4 yrs.	37	10.8 mos.
Maxillary	Female	22	6. 3	21	7. 2	21	11.7
Maxillary	Total	65	6. 5	58	7. 3	58	11.1
Mandibular	Male	44	6. 2	40	7. 7	40	17.7
Mandibular	Female	22	5.11	18	7. 4	18	15.9
Mandibular	Total	66	6.1	58	7. 6	58	17.1

Source: Sato Institute of Dental Research

This table shows the average age at the beginnings and completion of occlusal surface eruption of the 1st molar. The average length of time required for complete eruption is also given.

Table 2. Second Molar Eruption Start Time and Occlusal Surface Eruption Completion Time.

Jaws	Period Sex	Eruption Start Time N	Average	Completion N	Average	Period N	Average
Maxillary	Male	12	11.10 yrs.	12	12. 6 yrs.	12	8. 7 mos.
Maxillary	Female	25	12. 2	20	12.11	20	7. 8
Maxillary	Total	37	12. 1	32	12. 9	32	8. 1
Mandibular	Male	17	11. 5	14	12. 4	14	12. 1
Mandibular	Female	23	11. 7	13	13. 1	13	18. 2
Mandibular	Total	40	11. 6	27	12. 8	27	15. 0

Source: Sato Institute of Dental Research

This table shows the average age at the beginnings and completion of occlusal surface eruption of the second molar. It shows that the averge length of time for completion of eruption: 8.1 months for the maxillary and 15.0 months for the mandibular.

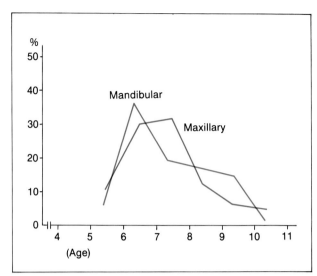

Fig. 32. Distribution of First Molar Occlusal Surface Eruption Times. (Source: Sato Institute of Dental Research)

The age distribution for completion of occlusal surface eruption of the first molar. Eruption is completed in some children before the age of six, while others may not experience complete eruption until they are over 10 years old.

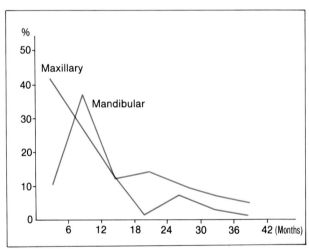

Fig. 33. Distribution of First Molar occlusal Surface Eruption Periods. (Source: Sato Institute of Dental Research)

The age distribution for the length of time required for complete eruption of the occlusal surface of the first molar. Some children experience complete eruption in less than 3 months, while other children may experience an eruption period lasting for over 36 months.

5 MAXILLARY CENTRAL INCISORS

Maxillary Central Incisors

The average eruption time for the maxillary central incisors is approximately 7 years of age. They erupt from the incisal edge and at a faster pace than that seen in other permanent teeth. They erupt into the positions of the primary central incisors, but with a more labial inclination. Gingivitis occurs more frequently around the marginal area, in relation to tooth eruption, because of the increased tendency toward food accumulation.

─────── **Notes on Anatomical Form and Occlusal Surfaces** ───────

1. In many cases, the labial surface has a trapezoidal or rectangular outer form.

2. The corners on the mesial and distal edges are rounded, especially those on the distal edge.

ERUPTION OF RIGHT MAXILLARY CENTRAL INCISOR
(Girl, age 7 years at start of eruption)

NOTE: The (a) photos are from the labial side and the (b) photos from the lingual side.
The eruption of the incisors and canines is observed from both the labial side and from the incisal edge (including the lingual side) for a more detailed view. The photographs for these teeth are shown in labial-side/lingual-side pairs, and each pair was photographed on the same occasion.

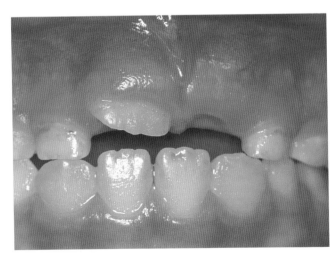

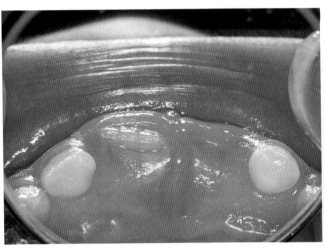

Fig. 1-a. One week after exfoliation of the primary right maxillary central incisor, the permanent one begins to erupt. The center of the gingiva appears depressed, following the exfoliation of the primary incisor.

Fig. 1-b. From below, the emerging central edge can be seen, along with gingival swelling on the labial and lingual sides.

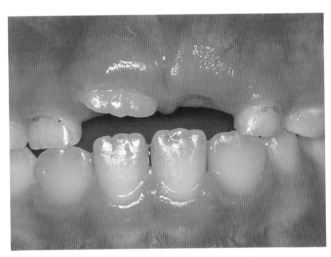

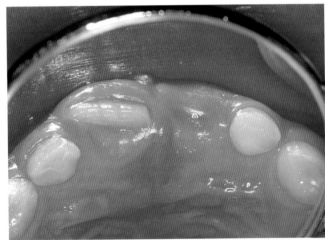

Fig. 2-a. 10 days later: the mesial corner has erupted.

Fig. 2-b. The incisal edge is distally inclined.

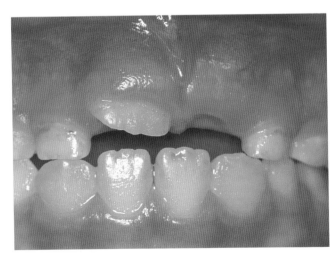

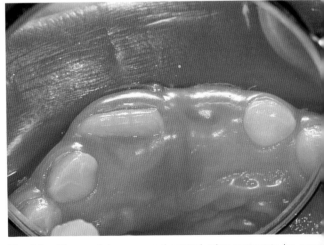

Fig. 3-a. 2 weeks later: although the tooth is erupting quickly, the distal corner has still not completely erupted.

Fig. 3-b. The mesial corner and central edge appear to be completely erupted; but the distal corner is not.

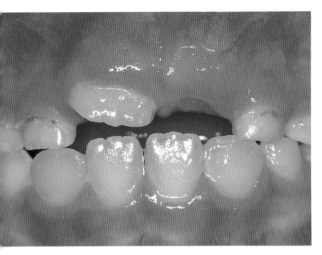

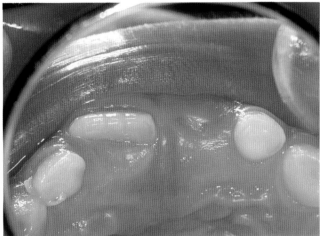

g. 4-a. 3 weeks after the initial eruption, only a slight bit of the distal corner has still not erupted.

Fig. 4-b. The distal corner has still not fully erupted.

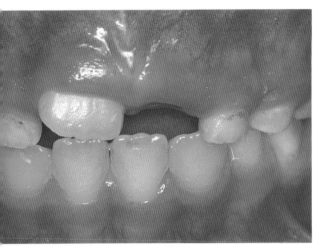

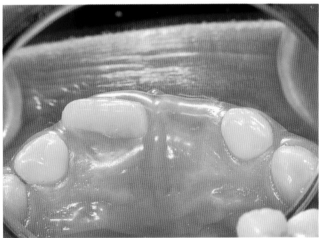

g. 5-a. 4 weeks later: the distal corner has fully erupted.

Fig. 5-b. Eruption has progressed to include all of the distal corner.

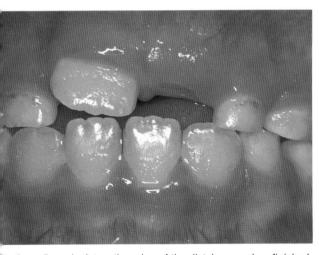

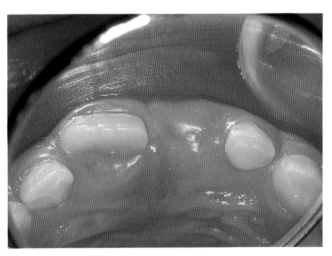

g. 6-a. 5 weeks later: the edge of the distal corner has finished erupting to complete the emergence process, about 1 month after initial eruption.

Fig. 6-b. Emergence of the central edge is complete.

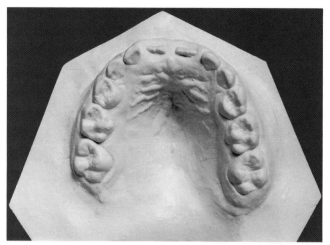

Fig. 7. At 6 years, 4 months: during normal replacement of the primary teeth, the permanent central incisors erupt into the primary incisors' positions. There is however, a tendency to erupt in a twisted fashion, in which the crown's distal side projects labially (No. 199).

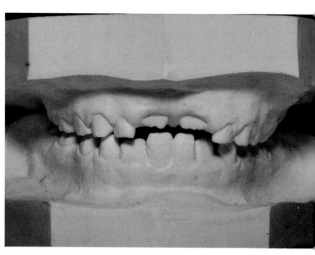

Fig. 8. At 6 years, 4 months: the maxillary permanent central incisors have not yet reached the occlusal line of the mandibular central incisors (No. 199).

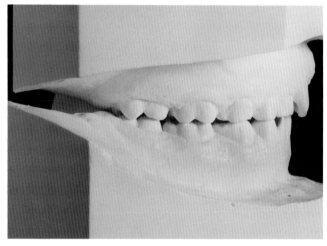

Fig. 9. At 6 years, 8 months: 4 months later, both the right and left maxillary central incisors have erupted to the labial side of the primary arch and the right maxillary central incisor has rotated distally (No. 199).

Clinical Memo

1. Eruption stages 1 and 2: much influenced by the primary incisors, the permanent central incisors usually erupt in their predecessors' positions, although in some cases they will protrude on the labial side. The incisal edges erupt quickly, having sharp angles that are conducive to eruption (first 2 weeks of eruption).

2. Eruption stage 3: nearly the entire edge has emerged, but the distal edge has not yet erupted completely (3rd or 4th week of eruption).

3. Eruption stage 4: the distal edge has erupted to complete the incisor's emergence process. The incisors will appear much bigger on the labial side than the surrounding primary teeth.

6 MANDIBULAR CENTRAL INCISORS

Mandibular Central Incisors

The average eruption time for mandibular central incisors is approximately 6 years of age and eruption starts at the incisal edge. These have been observed to erupt with various inclinations, such as the same inclination as primary incisors, a more lingual inclination of the mesial side, or a more labial inclination of the distal side.

Notes on Anatomical Form and Occlusal Surfaces

1. The labial side may show an oblong or U-shaped outer form.
2. The three developmental lobes of the central incisors are the same in the maxillary and mandibular teeth: the mesial, central, and distal development lobes.
3. The mesial and distal incisal angles are both about 85 degrees.
4. The incisal edge is a nearly straight line from the mesial to distal corners.

ERUPTION OF LEFT MANDIBULAR CENTRAL INCISOR
(Girl, age 5 years, 10 months at start of eruption)

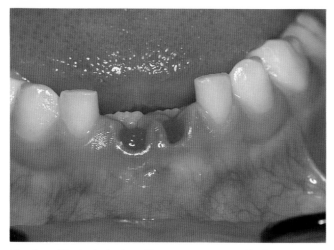

Fig. 1-a. The incisal edge of the permanent central incisor emerges between the primary lateral incisor.

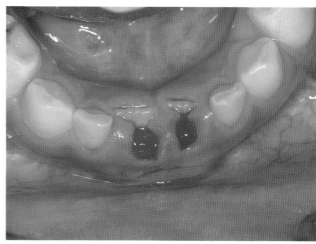

Fig. 1-b. The central incisor erupts lingually as it begins to emerge

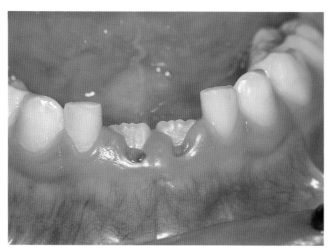

Fig. 2-a. 1 week later (11 days after initial eruption): the mesial corner of the incisal edge has erupted; the distal corner is still erupting.

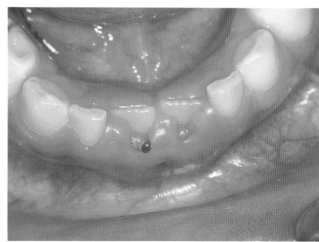

Fig. 2-b. The distal incisal edge is still erupting.

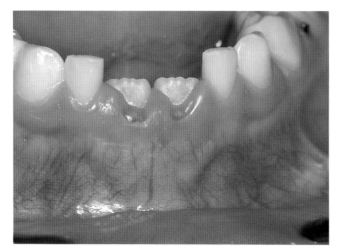

Fig. 3-a. 2 weeks later: the incisal edge is slowly erupting and the distal corner can be seen gradually rising above the gingiva.

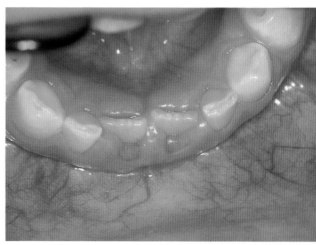

Fig. 3-b. The distal corner is now emerging.

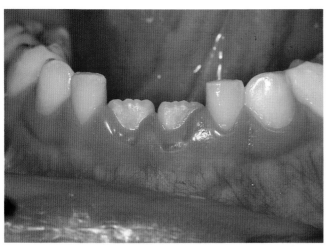

Fig. 4-a. 3 weeks later: eruption of the distal corner is almost complete.

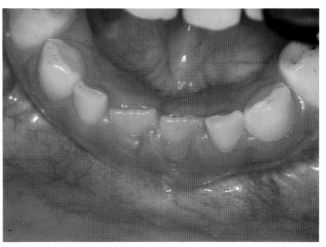

Fig. 4-b. The central incisor shifts labially as it erupts.

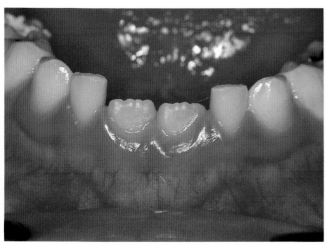

Fig. 5-a. 5 weeks (about 1 month) later: the left central incisor has erupted further and the distal corner has now clearly emerged.

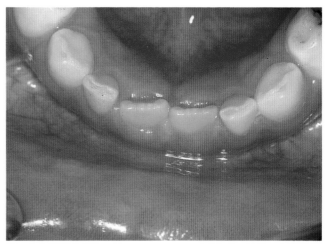

Fig. 5-b. Further eruption, including the distal corner.

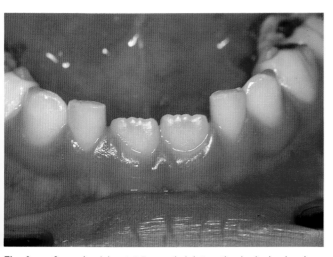

Fig. 6-a. 6 weeks (about 1.5 months) later: the incisal edge has erupted completely.

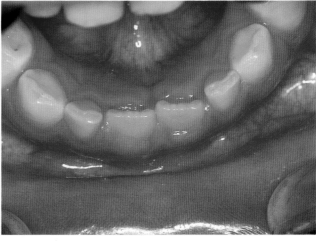

Fig. 6-b. Eruption is complete, from mesial to distal corners.

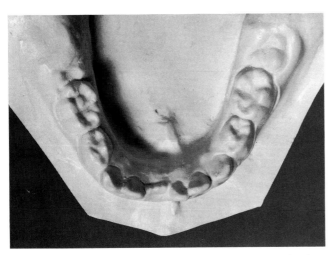

Fig. 7. At 5 years, 4 months: the right mandibular central incisor has fully emerged (No. 199).

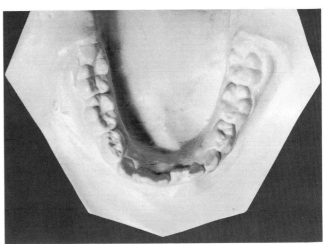

Fig. 8. At 5 years, 6 months: the left mandibular central incisor has begun to erupt. The left and right mandibular central incisors erupt simultaneously or in close succession. In this case, the right mandibular central incisor's incisal edge has already finished erupting (No. 199).

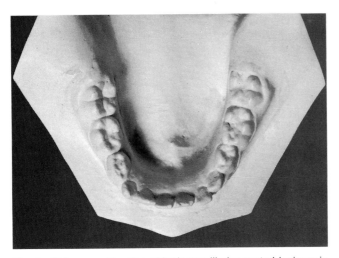

Fig. 9. At 6 years: Eruption of both mandibular central incisors is complete (No. 199).

Clinical Memo

1. Eruption stages 1 and 2: unlike the maxillary central incisors, the mandibular central incisors tend to erupt on the lingual side of their primary predecessors, and, in some cases, eruption begins even before the primary central incisors have fallen out. They usually erupt from the middle of their incisal edge and, in many cases, both the mesial and distal corners of the incisal edge erupt simultaneously (First 2 weeks of eruption).

2. Eruption stages 3 and 4: eruption of the distal corner of the incisal edge was somewhat retarded, and it is during stages 3 and 4 that they also erupt fully. The two mandibular central incisors gradually shift from the lingual side toward the labial side and end up aligned with the primary lateral incisors (3rd to 6th week of eruption).

7 MAXILLARY LATERAL INCISORS

Maxillary Lateral Incisors

The average eruption time for maxillary lateral incisors is approximately 8 years of age, and eruption begins from the incisal edge. This eruption period is longer than that of the maxillary central incisors, due to the influence of the anatomical form of the round distal incisal edge.

─────── **Notes on Anatomical Form and Occlusal Surfaces** ───────

1. While the lateral incisors have generally trapezoidal forms similar to central incisors, they are, overall, rounder.

2. Their outer form is similar to that of the central incisors only with rounder distal corners and, in some cases, a tendency toward degeneration.

ERUPTION OF MAXILLARY LATERAL INCISOR
(Girl, age 7 years at start of eruption)

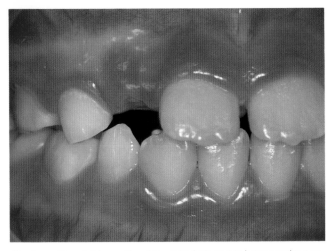

Fig. 1-a. The right maxillary lateral incisor erupts between the permanent central incisor and the primary canine, with eruption beginning one week after loss of the primary lateral incisor.

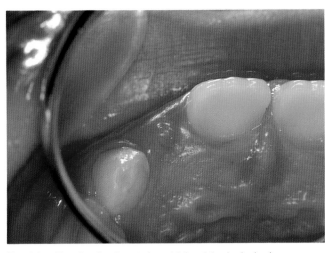

Fig. 1-b. Eruption begins at the middle of the incisal edge.

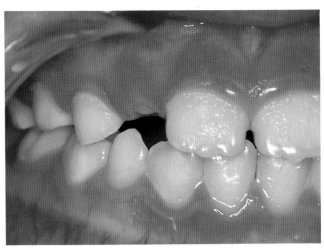

Fig. 2-a. 3 weeks later: the tooth erupts gradually.

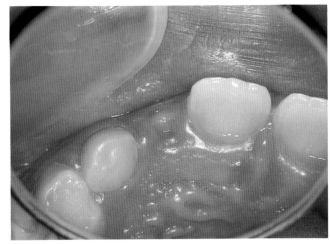

Fib. 2-b. The middle of the incisal edge emerges slowly.

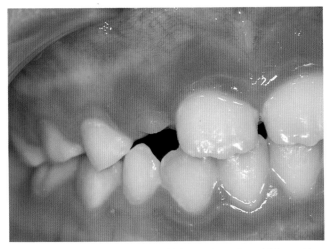

Fig. 3-a. 4 weeks (almost 1 month) later: the entire middle section of the incisal edge can be seen.

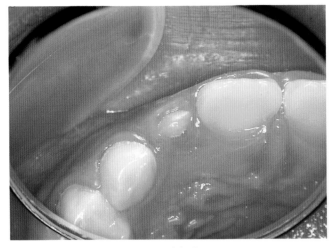

Fig. 3-b. Eruption has progressed further.

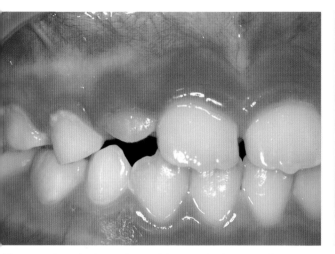

Fig. 4-a. 6 weeks later: the mesial corner is also emerging.

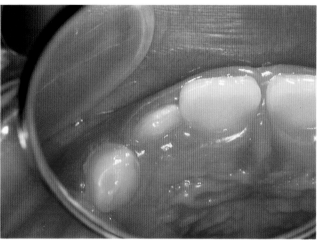

Fig. 4-b. On the incisal edge, only the distal corner remains covered.

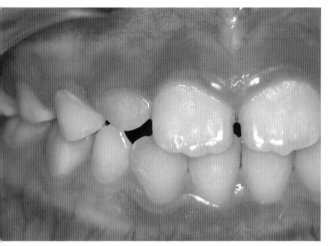

Fig. 5-a. 8 weeks later: the distal corner is also erupting.

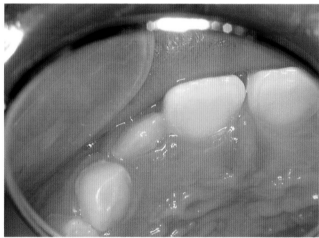

Fig. 5-b. The distal corner has not fully erupted.

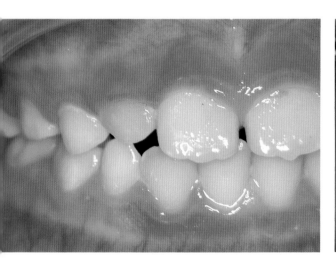

Fig. 6-a. 9 weeks (2 months) later: all of the incisal edge, including the distal corner, has fully erupted.

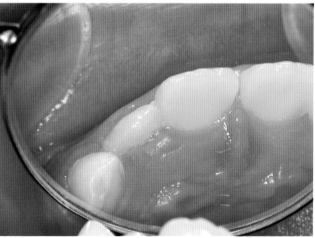

Fig. 6-b. The entire incisal edge has erupted.

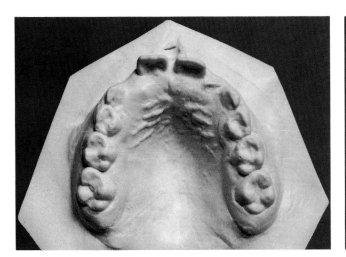

Fig. 7. At 7 years, 2 months: the left lateral incisor is slightly notated (No. 199).

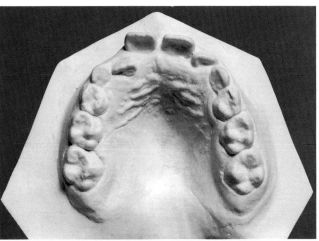

Fig. 8. At 7 years, 4 months: 2 months later, almost the entire incisal edge of the left lateral incisor has erupted. The right lateral incisor has erupted palatally (No. 199).

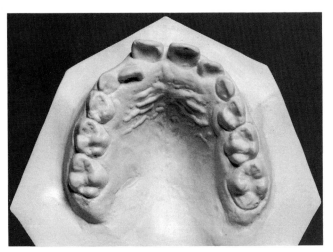

Fig. 9. At 7 years, 6 months: 2 months later, both of the maxillary lateral incisors have fully erupted. The left one has shifted labially to a position alongside the permanent central incisors, but the right one is still in the process of shifting (No. 199).

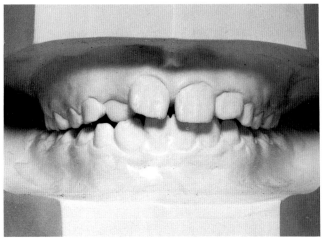

Fig. 10. At 7 years, 10 months: the right lateral incisor is twisted toward the mouth in a reversed occlusion pattern (No. 199).

Clinical Memo

1. There are some cases in which the shape of the maxillary lateral incisors is changed and other cases in which they erupt lingually or palatally. Eruption begins from the middle of the incisal edge.

2. In the same way, the mandibular lateral incisors have an even larger mesial/distal diameter than the mandibular central incisors, and, therefore, they sometimes rotate or twist lingually as they erupt. Eruption begins from the middle of the incisal edge.

8 MANDIBULAR LATERAL INCISORS

Mandibular Lateral Incisors

The average eruption time for mandibular lateral incisors is approximately 7 years of age and eruption begins at the incisal edge. The transition from gingival emergence to full eruption of the incisal edge is similar to that of the maxillary lateral incisors. It has been observed that these erupt in the normal position in the spaced type of the primary dentition and erupt with more lingual inclination in the closed type, which results in a crowding of teeth.

Notes on Anatomical Form and Occlusal Surfaces

1. They have a larger shape than the mandibular central incisors.
2. Development of the distal angle of the incisal edge is weak in comparison to that of the mesial corner, and the distal angle is also rounder.
3. The mandibular lateral incisors erupt, beginning with the middle of the incisal edge or the mesial corner.

ERUPTION OF RIGHT MANDIBULAR LATERAL INCISOR
(Girl, age 6 years, 6 months at start of eruption)

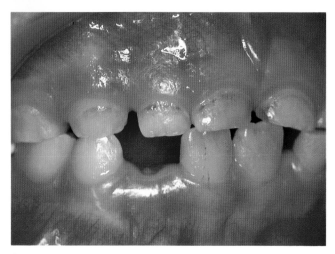

Fig. 1-a. 2 weeks after the primary lateral incisor was exfoliated, the middle of the incisal edge of the permanent lateral appears between the permanent central incisor and the primary canine.

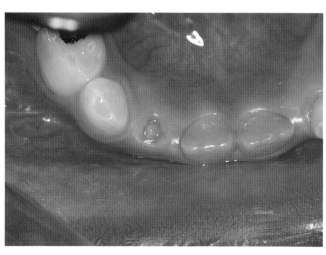

Fig. 1-b. Eruption of the occlusal surface begins at the middle of the incisal edge.

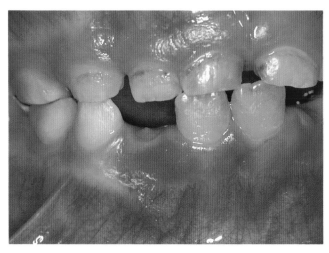

Fig. 2-a. 1 week later: the permanent lateral incisor erupts in the same position as its primary predecessor.

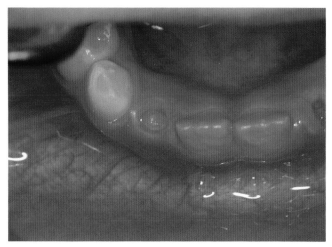

Fig. 2-b. Eruption occurs normally, within the row of mandibular teeth.

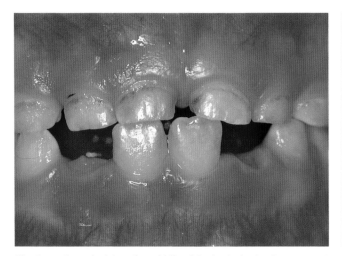

Fig. 3-a. 2 weeks later: the middle of the incisal edge has erupted further.

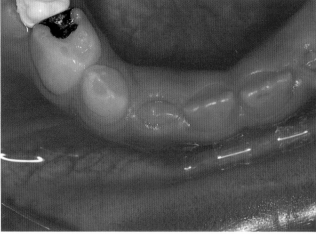

Fig. 3-b. Further eruption of the incisal edge can be seen.

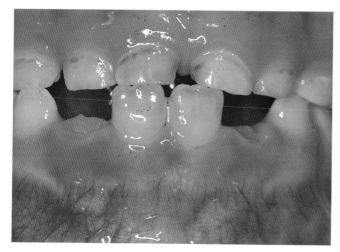

Fig. 4-a. 3 weeks later: eruption has progressed so that the general form of the incisal edge can be seen. The left mandibular lateral incisor has also begun to erupt.

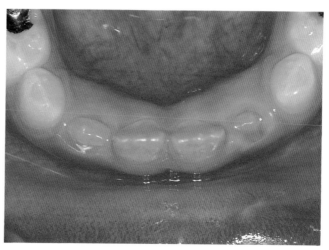

Fig. 4-b. The greater width of the lateral incisors over the central incisors can be seen as the lateral incisors erupt.

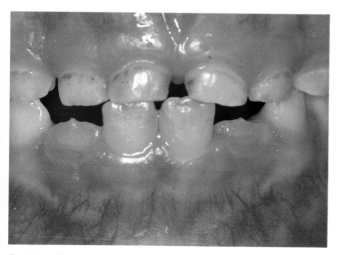

Fig. 5-a. 5 weeks (about 1 month) later: the mesial corner has erupted.

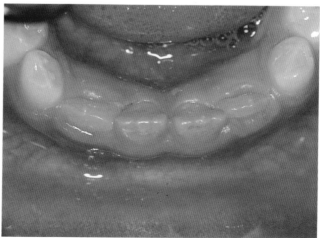

Fig. 5-b. The mesial corner has erupted, but the distal corner is still partially covered.

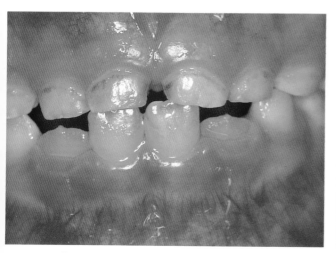

Fig. 6-a. 6 weeks (about 1.5 months) later: the distal corner has also erupted, completing the eruption of the incisal edge.

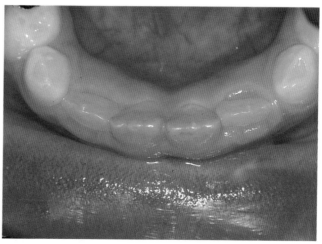

Fig. 6-b. The entire incisal edge, including the distal corner, has erupted.

Eruption of Incisors

The maxillary and mandibular central and lateral incisors all generally erupt in the same place as the primary dentition that preceded them. However, such factors as the development of the primary dentition and the presence or absence of developmental leeway can lead to abnormal positioning of the permanent incisors.

The eruption of incisors is easily influenced by both hereditary factors and environmental factors such as caries. In addition, sometimes, when the maxillary central incisors erupt, adjunct teeth usually closes such a gap. The mandibular central incisors erupt on the lingual side of the gingival cavities left by their primary prede-

cessors, and over the next several months, drift labially to close these cavities. Like the mandibular central incisors, the mandibular lateral incisors sometimes erupt with a lingual orientation and gradually shift to the correct position over a period of several months. Due to their similarity, the left and right incisors tend to erupt at the same time or in close succession. The maxillary lateral incisors often erupt in normal positions but sometimes are inclined or twisted toward the oral cavity. In cases where they are heavily twisted toward the oral cavity, reversed occlusion can result. Therefore, in such cases, care should be taken.

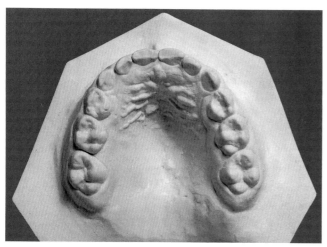

Fig. 7. At 7 years, 4 months: as they begin to erupt, the mesial side of the right lateral incisor is lingually twisted and the left lateral incisor is lingually rotated. Both lateral incisors erupt from the mesial corner to the middle of the incisal edge and finally to the distal corner (No. 199).

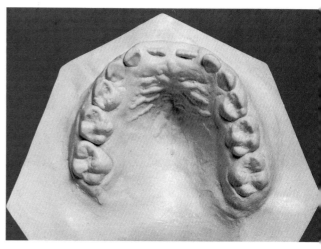

Fig. 8. At 7 years, 6 months: the distal corners have also erupted along with the rest of the incisal edge of the right lateral incisor. There is no change in the lingual twist of the left lateral incisor, nor in the rotation (No. 199).

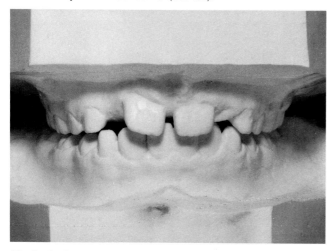

Fig. 9. At 7 years, 4 months: occlusion has not been attained between the maxillary and mandibular incisors. The maxillary left lateral incisor is twisted (No. 199).

Clinical Memo

1. The manbidular lateral incisors have an even larger mesial/distal diameter than the mandibular central incisors, and, therefore, they sometimes rotate or twist lingually as they erupt. Eruption begins from the middle of the incisal edge.

9 MAXILLARY CANINES

Maxillary Canines

The average eruption time for maxillary canines is approximately 10 to 11 years of age and eruption begins from the incisal edge. These teeth take longer to erupt than maxillary incisors, due to the round mesial and distal corners of their crowns. They erupt with more labial inclination than other permanent teeth and often tend to migrate toward the labial or facial side.

--- **Notes on Anatomical Form and Occlusal Surfaces** ---

1. The outer form is a pentagonal shape, and the crown has a wide diameter.
2. The incisal edge has a small tip that indicates the conspicuous development of the middle developmental lobe.
3. The incisal edge is divided into mesial and distal incisal edges, and the latter is the longer of the two.

ERUPTION OF RIGHT MAXILLARY CANINE
(Girl, age 9 years, 7 months, at the start of eruption)

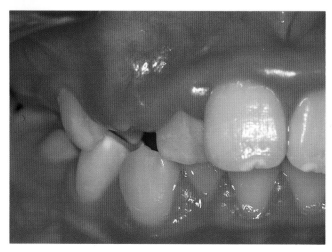

Fig. 1-a. The tip of the canine tooth can be seen emerging between the lateral incisor and the first premolar. The gingiva appears to be congested with blood.

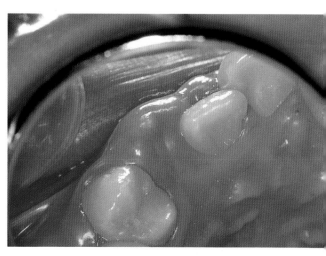

Fig. 1-b. The lateral incisor and first premolar have already erupted, and the canine erupts between them from the labial side.

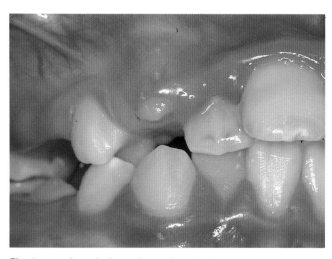

Fig. 2-a. 2 weeks later: the canine slowly erupts, beginning with the tip.

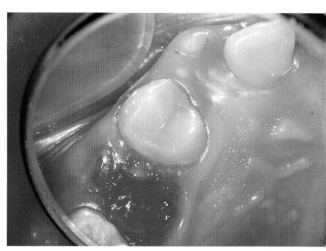

Fig. 2-b. As the eruption slowly progressed, the primary second molar exfoliated.

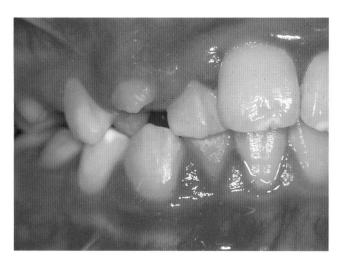

Fig. 3-a. 6 weeks (about 1.5 months) later: eruption from the tip progresses to include the mesial and distal incisal edges.

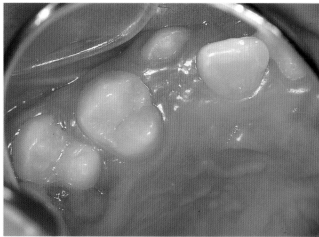

Fig. 3-b. The canine shifts on the labial side and exposes the lingual ridge.

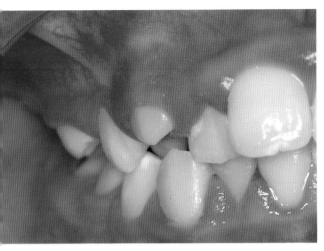

Fig. 4-a. 10 weeks later: eruption continues from the tip to the mesial and distal incisal edge.

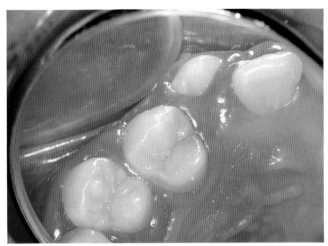

Fig. 4-b. Eruption of mesial and distal edges continues.

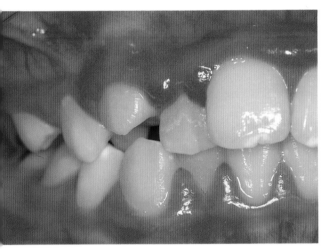

Fig. 5-a. 13 weeks (about 3 months) later: eruption progresses almost to the mesial and distal corners.

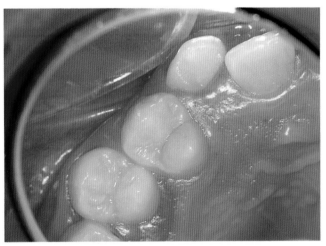

Fig. 5-b. The mesial corner erupts well before the distal corner.

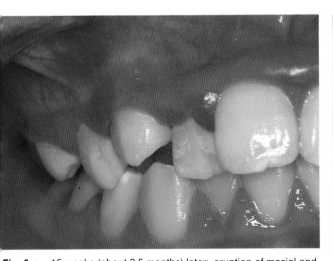

Fig. 6-a. 15 weeks (about 3.5 months) later: eruption of mesial and distal corners continues, and overall eruption is almost complete.

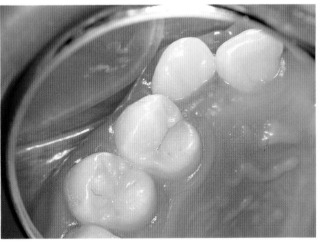

Fig. 6-b. Eruption is complete with the full emergence of the mesial and distal corners.

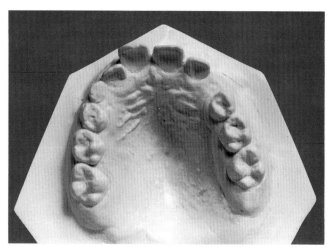

Fig. 7. At 9 years: the tip of the canine begins to emerge from the gingiva (No. 199).

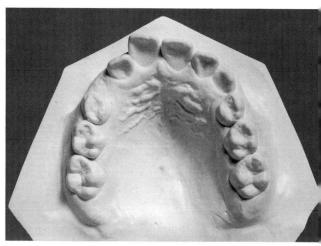

Fig. 8. At 9 years, 2 months: most of the incisal section, including the mesial and distal corners, emerges at a relatively fast pace. This case also shows the gap left by the right primary molar (No. 199).

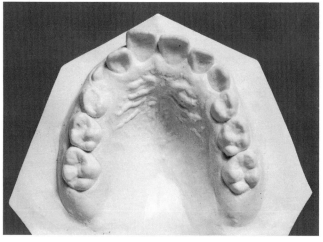

Fig. 9. At 9 years, 4 months: eruption of the left canine's incisal edge is complete with the emergence of the mesial and distal corners. The eruption of the right canine is delayed (No. 199).

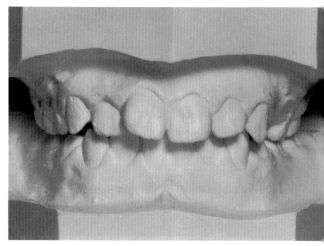

Fig. 10. At 9 years, 8 months: the teeth have not yet occluded.

Clinical Memo

1. Eruption stages 1 and 2: the canine teeth are influenced by their primary predecessors. They erupt between the lateral incisors and the first premolars and can sometimes be late in erupting. There are a relatively large number of cases in which the canine rotates to the labial side. Eruption begins from the tip (1st to 6th week of eruption).

2. Eruption stages 3 and 4: eruption, as far as the mesial and distal corners, requires a long period, and it is during this period that the canines shift to meet the row of permanent teeth (7th to 15th week of eruption).

10 MANDIBULAR CANINES

Mandibular Canines

The average eruption time for the mandibular canines is approximately 9 to 10 years of age, and eruption begins from the incisal edge. Their anatomical form is very similar to that of the maxillary canine. The mandibular canines, more than other teeth, usually erupt in proper alignment. If there isn't enough space, eruption is generally toward the labial side of the dental arch.

—————— **Notes on Anatomical Form and Occlusal Surfaces** ——————

1. The mandibular canines resemble their maxillary counterparts but have smaller crowns.

2. The mandibular canines appear between the incisors and the premolars.

ERUPTION OF LEFT MANDIBULAR CANINE
(Girl, age 9 years, 3 months, at the start of eruption)

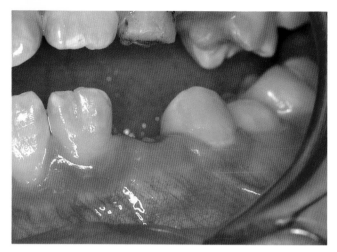

Fig. 1-a. The tip of the canine's incisal edge appears in the gingiva cavity between the lateral incisor and the first primary molar.

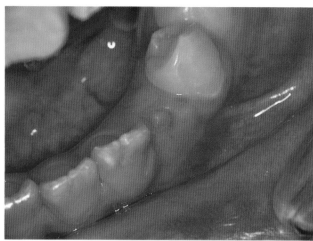

Fig. 1-b. The tip of the canine appears.

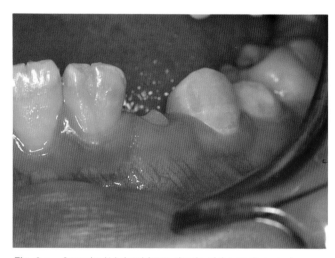

Fig. 2-a. 2 weeks (14 days) later: the tip of the canine can be seen clearly.

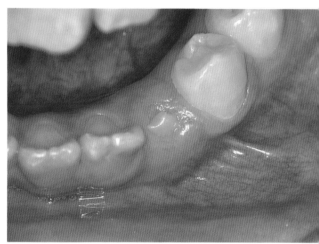

Fig. 2-b. The tip and part of the lingual ridge are visible.

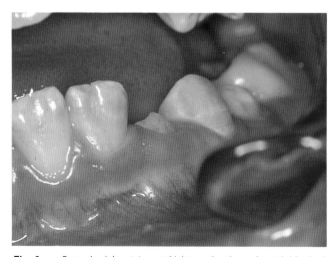

Fig. 3-a. 5 weeks (about 1 month) later: the tip and mesial incisal edge have emerged.

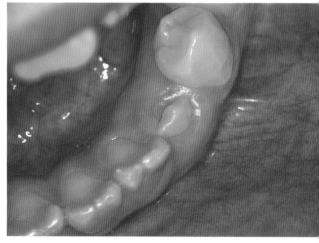

Fig. 3-b. Eruption gradually progresses to include the mesial and distal incisal edges. The tooth erupts in a normal position between the lateral incisor and first premolar.

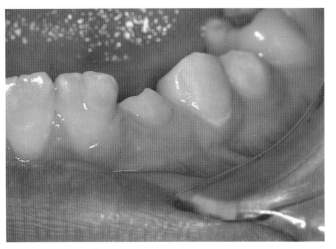

Fig. 4-a. 8 weeks (about 2 months) later: eruption has progressed almost to the mesial and distal corners.

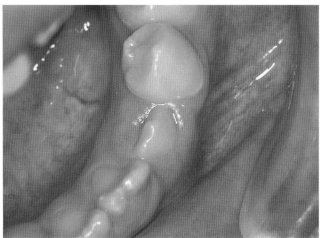

Fig. 4-b. Both the mesial and distal corners are about to emerge.

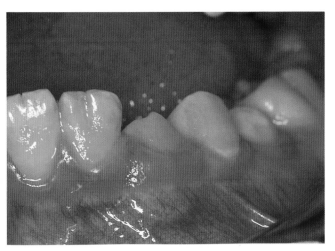

Fig. 5-a. 10 weeks (about 2 months) later: part of the mesial and distal corners can now be seen.

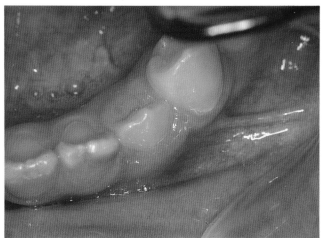

Fig. 5-b. The canine appears wider as the mesial and distal corners begin to emerge.

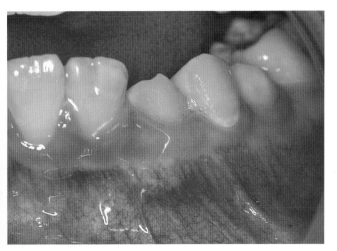

Fig. 6-a. 12 weeks (about 3 months) later: both the mesial and distal corners have emerged, and eruption of the entire incisal edge is complete.

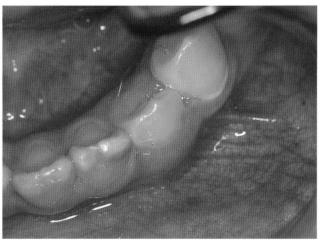

Fig. 6-b. The entire canine crown, including the tip and corners, is in a normal position. Eruption is complete.

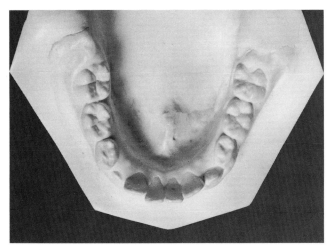

Fig. 7. At 8 years, 4 months: the right mandibular canine begins to erupt from the tip of the incisal edge. This occurred 2 months after the primary canine fell out (No. 199).

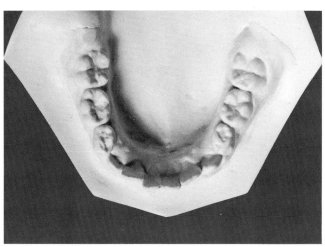

Fig. 8. At 8 years, 6 months: eruption has progressed to include the mesial and part of the distal corner. The right canine has also begun to erupt (No. 199).

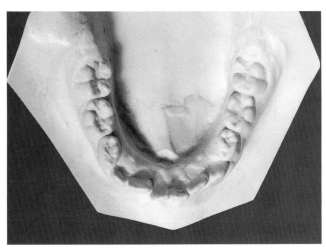

Fig. 9. At 8 years, 8 months: the left canine has erupted completely. The right canine is still erupting (No. 199).

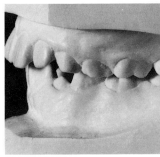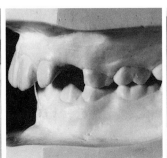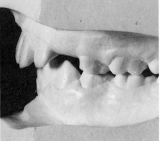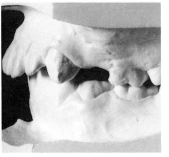

| 8 yrs., 2 mos. | 8 yrs., 4 mos. | 8 yrs., 8 mos. | 9 yrs., 8 mos. |

Fig. 10. Phases in the Occlusion of Maxillary and Mandibular Canines (No. 199).

Clinical Memo

1. Eruption stages 1 and 2: eruption begins from the tip of the incisal edge. The mandibular canines erupt into relatively normal positions and, during these stages, erupt until part of the mesial and distal corners can be seen (1st to 5th week of eruption).

2. Eruption stages 3 and 4: a relatively long period is required for the mesial and distal corners to erupt fully (6th to 12th week of eruption).

11 MAXILLARY FIRST PREMOLARS

Maxillary First Premolars

The average eruption age for maxillary first premolars is approximately 10 years. Occasionally, eruption begins as early as 8 years of age. Because these teeth have cusps on both the buccal and lingual sides, eruption takes longer than for the maxillary incisors.

The buccal cusp erupts first, followed by the lingual cusp. Usually, the maxillary first premolars erupt soon after the maxillary primary first molars have exfoliated, although eruption is sometimes delayed.

Notes on Anatomical Form and Occlusal Surfaces

1. The premolars have two cusps: a buccal cusp, which resembles the tip of the canine, and a lingual cusp.
2. The occlusal surface is an oval or hexagonal shape.
3. The occlusal surface ends with triangular ridges on the buccal side, and generally includes a central sulcus as well as mesial and distal grooves.

ERUPTION OF LEFT MAXILLARY FIRST PREMOLAR
(Girl, age 8 years, 9 months, at the start of eruption)

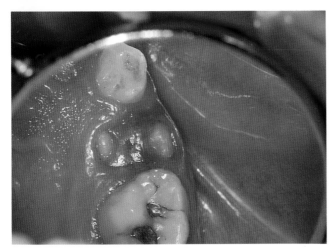

Fig. 1. The maxillary first premolar erupts first from the buccal cusps and then from the lingual cusp. It is possible for these cusps to begin erupting even before the primary tooth has exfoliated.

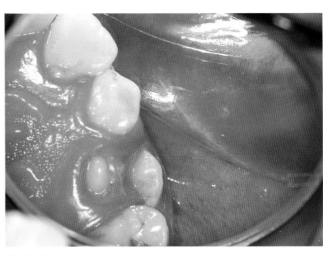

Fig. 2. 5 weeks (about 1 month) later: the cusps have erupted further, and the central sulcus is about to emerge. As of yet, it is still covered by gingiva.

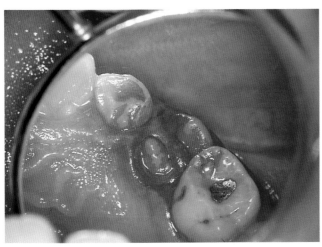

Fig. 3. 7 weeks later: the buccal and lingual cusps have erupted further and the gingiva covering the central sulcus is gradually receding. Fuchsine dye shows stains in the gingival area.

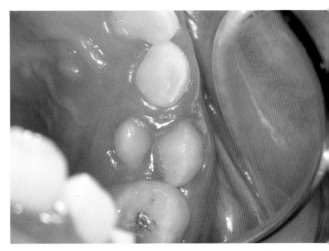

Fig. 4. 8 weeks later: most of the occlusal surface has erupted; however a small amount of gingiva still bridges the central sulcus.

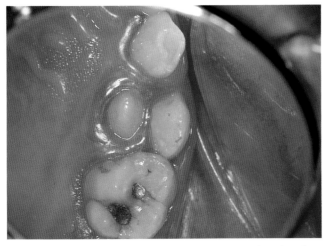

Fig. 5. 10 weeks (about 2 months) later: the occlusal surface has erupted further, although a thin thread of gingiva still bridges the central sulcus.

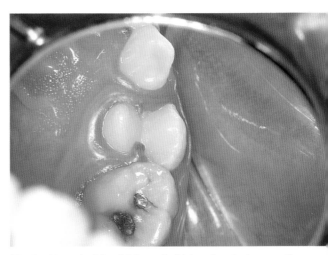

Fig. 6. 11 weeks (about 2.5 months) later: the gingiva over the central sulcus has separated but still covers the mesial and distal grooves.

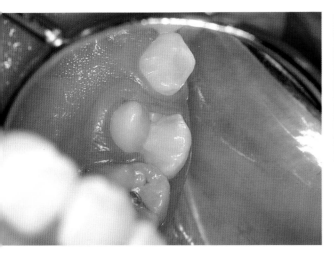

Fig. 7. 12 weeks later: the gingiva covering the mesial and distal grooves, has receded but still covers the mesial and distal ridges. (The use of a sealant to prevent caries is very effective at this stage.)

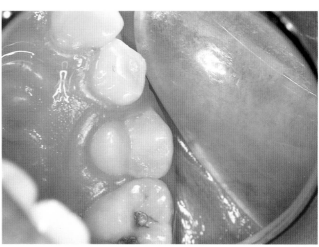

Fig. 8. 16 weeks (about 3.5 months) later: the gingiva, on the mesial and distal sides, has receded much further but still covers part of the mesial and distal ridges.

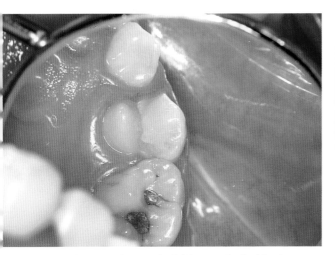

Fig. 9. 18 weeks later: the marginal ridges on both sides have not yet fully erupted.

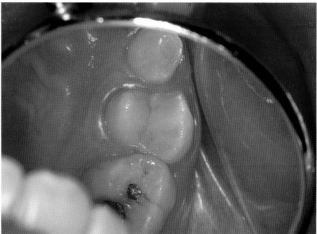

Fig. 10. 23 weeks (about 5 months) later: part of the ridge on the mesial edge remains covered.

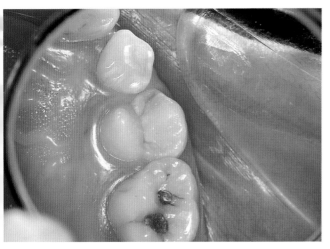

Fig. 11. 25 weeks (about 6 months) later: the occlusal surface has erupted completely.

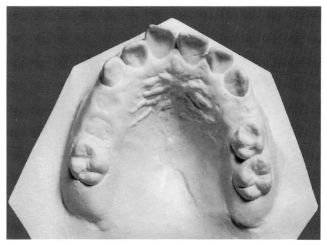

Fig. 12. At 10 years: the left maxillary first premolar begins erupting at its buccal cusp (No. 199).

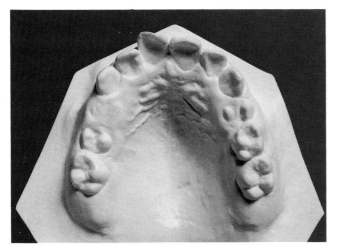

Fig. 13. At 10 years, 2 months: 2 months later, the lingual cusp has also begun to erupt (No. 199).

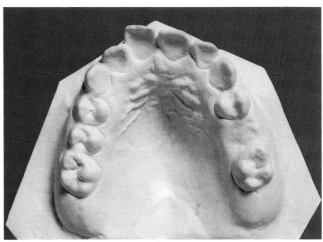

Fig. 14. At 10 years, 6 months: 6 months later, the occlusal surface has erupted completely (No. 199).

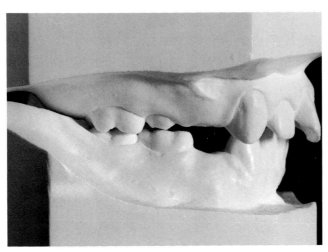

Fig. 15. At 10 years, 2 months: 2 months after the beginning of occlusal drift, the maxillary and mandibular dentition has not yet reached the occlusal line (No. 199).

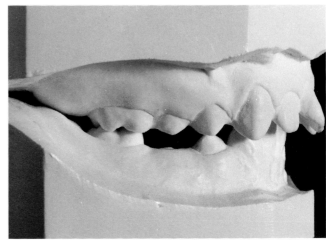

Fig. 16. At 10 years, 6 months: the occlusal drift now begins to show one-to-one contact between the maxillary and mandibular first premolars (No. 199).

Clinical Memo

1. Eruption stages 1 and 2: the first premolars erupt more quickly than the canines and second premolars. In normal cases, the buccal cusp of the first premolar erupts immediately after the exfoliation of its primary predecessor. In some cases, the first premolar's buccal and lingual cusps erupt simultaneously (1st to 5th week of eruption).

2. Eruption stage 3: the buccal cusps erupt further and nearly two-thirds of the occlusal surface becomes exposed. During this stage, the gingiva forms a bridge across the central sulcus. The gingiva edges can easily be contaminated and are difficult to clean (until about the 10th week of eruption).

3. Eruption stages 4 and 5: most of the occlusal surface is erupted, although most of the central groove is still covered by gingiva. Finally, the entire occlusal surface erupts; but, after this, a relatively long time is still required for full eruption of the tooth (until about the 25th week of eruption).

12 MANDIBULAR FIRST PREMOLARS

Mandibular First Premolars

The average eruption time for mandibular first premolars is approximately 9 to 10 years of age. They are similar to maxillary first premolars, in that they have cusps on both the buccal and lingual sides; however, their shape differs, in that their lingual cusps are not well developed. Eruption occurs at the buccal cusps, unlike the exfoliated primary mandibular first molars.

Notes on Anatomical Form and Occlusal Surfaces

1. Development of the lingual cusp is weak and this cusp is usually small.
2. The crown's outer form is an imperfect circular shape.
3. This tooth has a small occlusal surface which consists of a central sulcus and a triangular groove.

ERUPTION OF LEFT MANDIBULAR FIRST PREMOLAR
(Girl, age 10 years, 9 months, at the start of eruption)

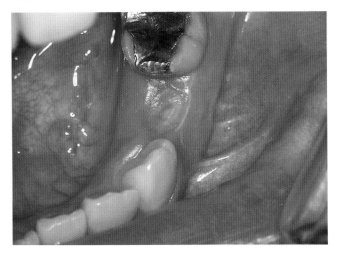

Fig. 1. The mandibular first premolar erupts in a position between the permanent canine and the primary second molar, emerging first from the buccal cusp.

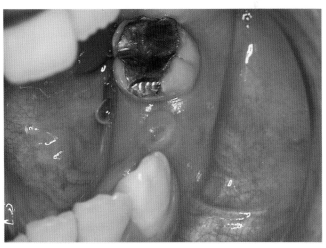

Fig. 2. 1 week later: the buccal cusp has erupted only a little further.

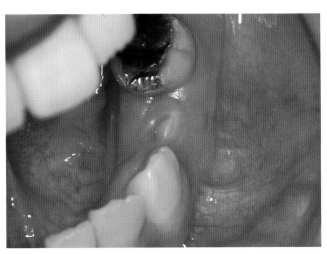

Fig. 3. 3 weeks later: the cusp slowly erupts.

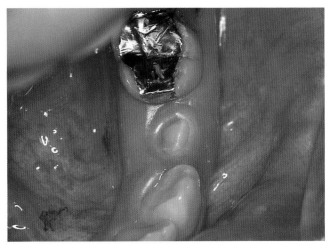

Fig. 4. 6 weeks (about one month) later: the buccal cusp and the mesial marginal ridge slope are emerging.

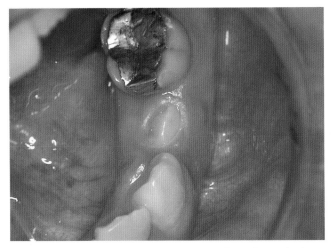

Fig. 5. 8 weeks (about two months) later: the buccal cusp is about one-third erupted, while the lingual cusp remains beneath the gingival surface, causing some swelling.

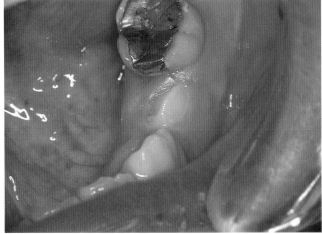

Fig. 6. 10 weeks later: the mesial groove of the buccal occlusal surface is emerging, although the lingual cusp still remains beneath the gingival surface.

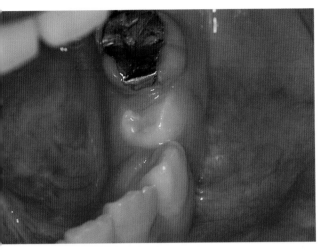

Fig. 7. 12 weeks later: the gingiva has receded rapidly, while nearly three-quarters of the crown has erupted from the mesial side to the lingual occlusal surface and from the mesial sulcus to the central groove.

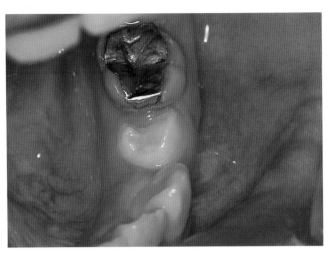

Fig. 8. 14 weeks later: eruption has progressed to the distobuccal corner and the gingiva now covers only the distal grooves and the distal marginal ridge.

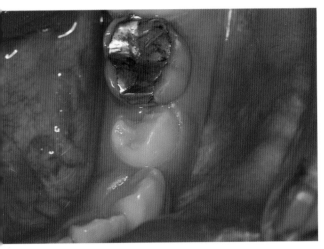

Fig. 9. 15 weeks (about 3.5 months) later: the small distal grooves can be seen, although gingiva still covers part of the distal marginal ridge.

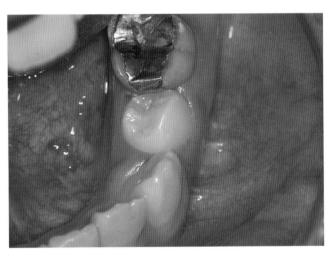

Fig. 10. 16 weeks (about 4 months) later: the gingiva has receded from the distolingual edge and the occlusal surface is now completely erupted.

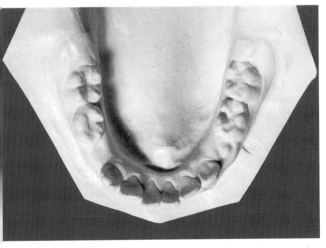

Fig. 11. At 10 years: eruption of the left mandibular first premolar begins at the buccal cusp (No. 199).

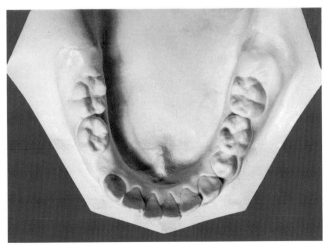

Fig. 12. At 10 years, 2 months: 2 months later, most of the occlusal surface, from the mesial edge to the buccal and lingual cusps, has erupted and only the small distal grooves and the distal edge remain covered by gingiva (No. 199).

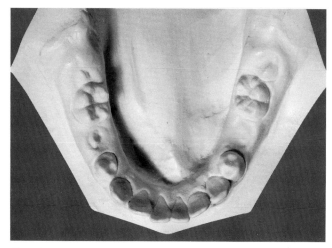

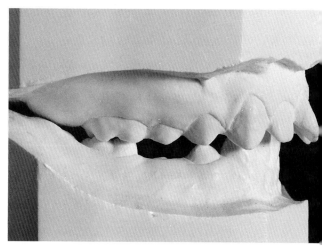

Fig. 13. At 10 years, 6 months: 6 months later, the occlusal surface is completely erupted (No. 199).

Fig. 14. At 10 years, 8 months: the maxillary first premolar finally touches the buccal cusp (No. 199).

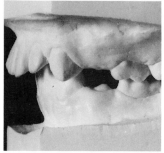
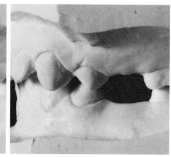
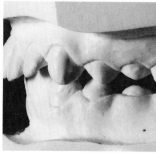

| 10 yrs. | 10 yrs., 2 mos. | 10 yrs., 6 mos. | 10 yrs., 8 mos |

Fig. 15. Phases in the Occlusion of Maxillary and Mandibular First Premolars (No. 199).

Clinical Memo

1. Eruption stages 1 and 2: the formation of the lingual cusp is marked by weak development; the result of this is that the lingual cusp takes a long time to emerge, even after the emergence of the buccal cusp. After the start of eruption, 3 to 8 weeks are required for eruption to progress form the emergence of the buccal cusp to that of about one-third of the occlusal surface (1st to 8th week of eruption).

2. Eruption stage 3: during this stage, the buccal and lingual cusps erupt further, as the gingiva recedes from the mesial edge and exposes about two-thirds of the occlusal surface. During this stage, the first premolars are easier to clean than the molars (6th to 13th week of eruption).

3. Eruption stages 4 and 5: the buccal cusp and nearly all of the occlusal surface has erupted, although the distal edge is still covered by gingiva. The transition from this stage to full eruption sometimes requires nearly a month (14th to 16th week of eruption).

13 MAXILLARY SECOND PREMOLARS

Maxillary Second Premolars

The average eruption time for maxillary second premolars is approximately 9 to 11 years of age. Their occlusal surfaces are similar to those of the maxillary first premolars, and there are two cusps (buccal and lingual) which are smaller than those of the maxillary first premolars.

These teeth erupt into positions between the maxillary first molars and the maxillary first premolars. Eruption may be malpositioned, however, to mesial drifting of the maxillary first molar, or premature loss of the primary molars. Generally, the buccal cusps erupt first, although occasionally both cusps will erupt at the same time.

Notes on Anatomical Form and Occlusal Surfaces

1. The maxillary second premolars are smaller than the first premolars.
2. The corners are rounded and the crown is generally round.
3. The central groove is shorter than that of the first premolar.

ERUPTION OF LEFT MAXILLARY SECOND PREMOLAR
(Girl, age 9 years, 10 months at the start of eruption)

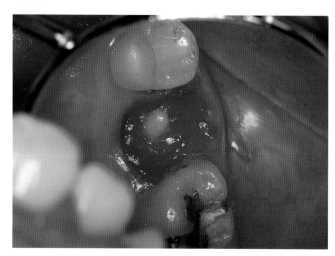

Fig. 1. The second premolar erupts form the lingual cusp in a position between the first premolar and the first molar. This occurs amid the blood-congested gingiva left by the exfoliated primary second molar.

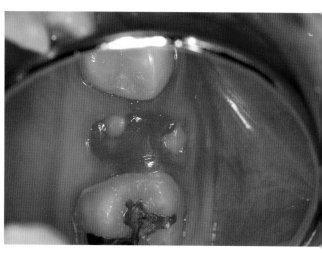

Fig. 2. 1 week later: still almost completely covered by gingiva only the lingual and buccal cusps have begun to emerge. The aftereffects of the primary second molar's exfoliation can still be seen.

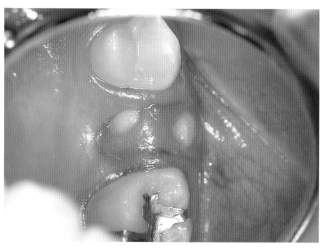

Fig. 3. 3 weeks later: the gingiva still covers most of the occlusal surface, and the lingual and buccal cusps are emerging slowly.

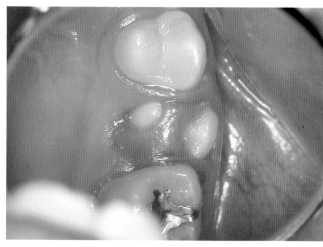

Fig. 4. 5 weeks (about 1 month) later: about one-third of the buccal cusp has erupted and the lingual cusp has erupted further. The peripheral gingiva appears congested with blood, and the large segment of gingiva over the central groove shows some swelling.

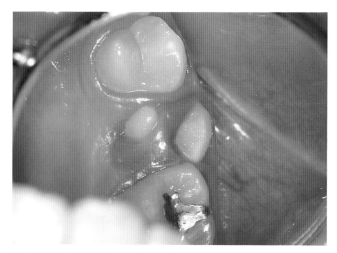

Fig. 5. 7 weeks (about 1.5 months) later: the buccal and lingual cusps gradually emerge between the first premolar and the first molar, with the buccal cusp emerging further.

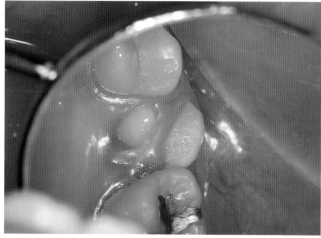

Fig. 6 9 weeks (two months) later: about two-thirds of the occlusal surface has erupted and the central groove remains covered by gingiva.

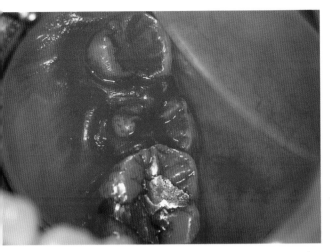

Fig. 7. Application of fuchsine dye shows staining strongest on the edges of the gingiva covering part of the occlusal surface.

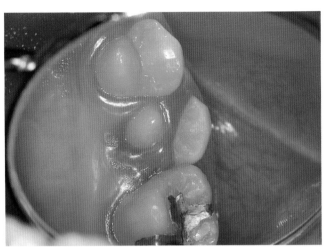

Fig. 8. 10 weeks (about two months) later: the gingiva is receding mesially and distally, exposing about four-fifths of the buccal occlusal surface and about one-third of the lingual occlusal surface.

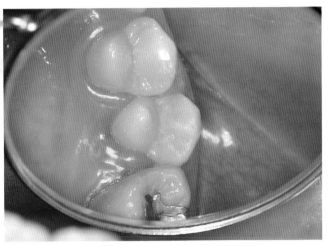

Fig. 9. 13 weeks (about 3 months) later: the occlusal surface appears to be fully erupted; however, the distal edge has not yet emerged completely.

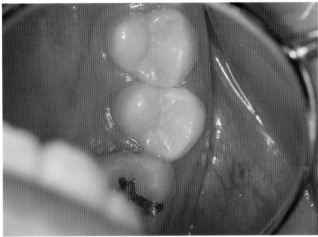

Fig. 10. 15 weeks (about 3.5 months) later: the occlusal surface has erupted completely.

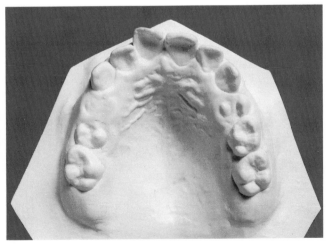

Fig. 11. At 10 years, 2 months: the right maxillary primary second molar exfoliated when the patient was 10 years old, and, two months later, we see most of the second premolar's occlusal surface has erupted, with the mesial and distal edges still covered by gingiva (No. 199).

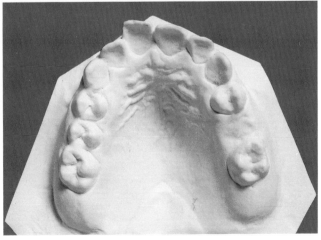

Fig. 12. At 10 years, 6 months: the occlusal surface has erupted completely (No. 199).

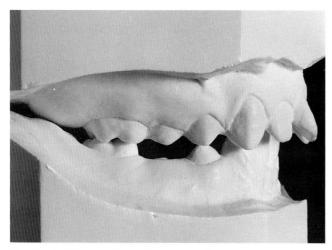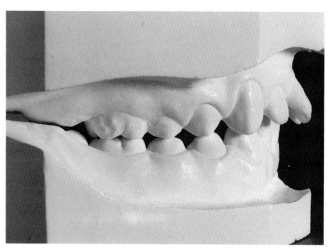

Fig. 13. At 10 years, 8 months: the mandibular second premolars exhibit slight buccal occlusion (No. 199).

Fig. 14. At 10 years, 10 months: the maxillary and mandibular second premolars are in mutual contact (No. 199).

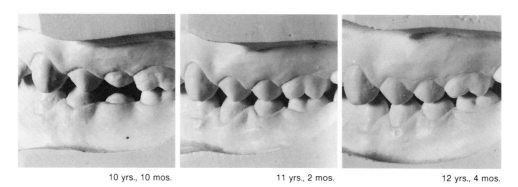

| 10 yrs., 10 mos. | 11 yrs., 2 mos. | 12 yrs., 4 mos. |

Fig. 15. Phases in the occlusion of maxillary and mandibular second premolars (No. 199).

Clinical Memo

1. Eruption stages 1 and 2: the maxillary second premolars erupt between the first premolars and the first molars, and their eruption time is influenced strongly by the primary second molar. Often, late exfoliation of this primary tooth will delay eruption of the second premolar. In some cases, lack of eruption leeway causes the second premolar to erupt into positions out of line with adjacent teeth. The buccal cusp typically erupts first. About 7 weeks after the start of eruption, the gingiva still covers the central groove and the mesial and lingual edges and the gingival edges are easily contaminated (1st to 7th week of eruption).

2. Eruption stage 3: At least two-thirds of the occlusal surface has erupted, and a narrow strip of gingiva still bridges the crown, from the mesial to distal edges, making this a difficult period for cleaning (8th to 10th week of eruption).

3. Eruption stages 4 and 5: nearly all of the occlusal surface has erupted, although a small amount of gingiva remains on the mesial and distal edges. Gradually, (in Stage 5) eruption becomes complete.

14 MANDIBULAR SECOND PREMOLARS

Mandibular Second Premolars

The average eruption time for mandibular second premolars is approximately 10 years of age. The lingual cusps of these teeth are well developed and are larger than those of the mandibular first premolars. The mesiodistal width of their crowns is smaller than that of the primary mandibular second molars, and eruption generally occurs in the normal position. If a mandibular first molar migrates mesially, due to caries in the primary second molar, this can cause mandibular second premolars to erupt at an angle. Generally, the buccal cusps erupt first, although occasionally both cusps erupt at the same time.

––––––– **Notes on Anatomical Form and Occlusal Surfaces** –––––––

1. The lingual cusps are well developed.
2. The outer form of the crown is roughly rectangular.
3. The occlusal surface consists of a central groove and triangular grooves.

ERUPTION OF RIGHT MANDIBULAR SECOND PREMOLAR
(Girl, age 10 years, 7 months at the start of eruption)

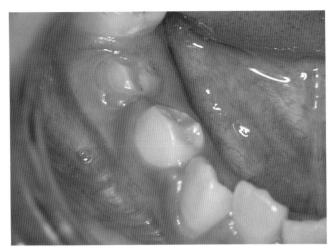

Fig. 1. The second premolar erupts in a position between the first premolar and the first molar, and about two-fifths of the lingual cusp can be seen. Once eruption has begun, it progresses quickly.

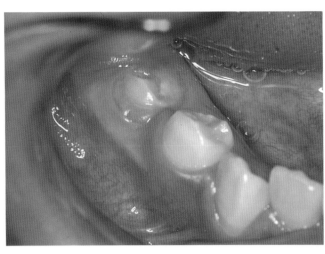

Fig. 2. 1 week later: the occlusal surface gradually erupts and the ridges on the occlusal surface can be seen.

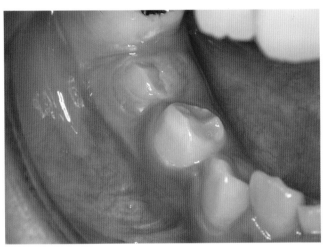

Fig. 3. 2 weeks later: the occlusal surface has erupted as far as the central groove.

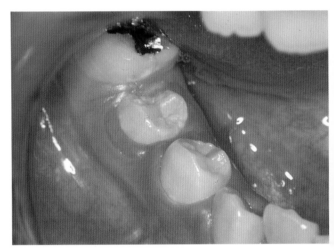

Fig. 4. 4 weeks later: eruption has progressed rapidly, to the point at which both cusps and most of the occlusal surface can be seen. Only a small amount of gingiva remains on the distal edge.

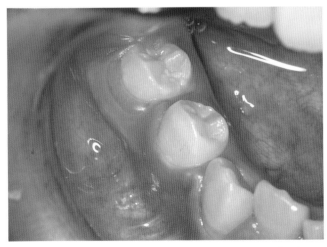

Fig. 5. 5 weeks (about 1 month) later: nearly all of the occlusal surface and the distal grooves have erupted. At this point, gaps can be seen on both the mesial and distal sides of the tooth.

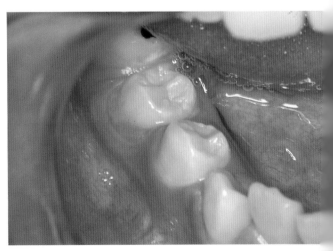

Fig. 6. 6 weeks later: almost all of the occlusal surface has erupted

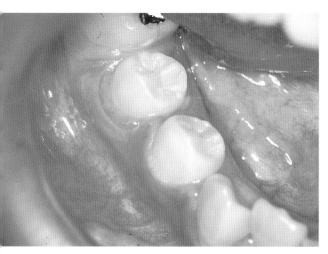

Fig. 7. The occlusal surface has erupted completely.

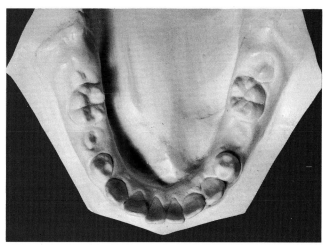

Fig. 8. At 10 years, 6 months: eruption of the right mandibular second premolar begins at the lingual cusp (No. 199).

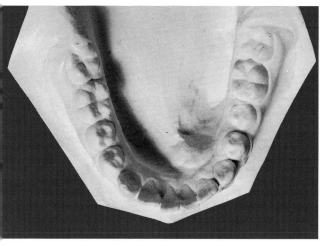

Fig. 9. At 10 years, 8 months: 2 months later, nearly all of the occlusal surface has erupted (No. 199).

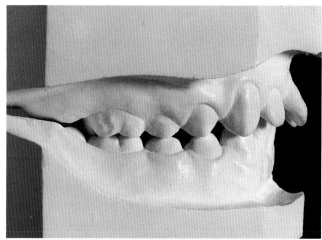

Fig. 10. At 10 years, 10 months: the mandibular and maxillary second premolars finally come into contact (No. 199).

Clinical Memo

1. Eruption stages 1 and 2: because the second premolars are smaller than the primary second molars, some extra space is left after the primary second molars are replaced, and the space aids in the normal eruption of the second premolars. However, caries in the primary teeth can cause the first molar to shift mesially. This should be noted when observing eruption of the second premolars, which generally erupt from the buccal cusps (1st to 3rd week of eruption).

2. Eruption stage 3: soon after eruption of the buccal cusps, the lingual cusps emerge rapidly, and overall eruption progresses to about two-thirds the occlusal surface. During this stage, cleaning of the occlusal surface is relatively easy (4th to 5th week of eruption).

3. Eruption stages 4 and 5: nearly all of the occlusal surface has erupted completely, although a small amount of gingiva remains on the mesial and distal edges (6th to 7th week of eruption).

Eruption of Canines, First Premolars, and Second Premolars

The canines, first premolars, and second premolars erupt between the first molars and the incisors at approximately 8 to 10 years of age, and they are characterized by the close proximity of their eruption periods. The primary molars are prone to caries, which in many cases disturbs root resorption, causes variations during the exfoliation period, and produces other hindrances to normal replacement of permanent teeth.

The role of the lateral teeth is to contribute to the formation of the row of permanent teeth; therefore, any variation in the lateral teeth's eruption order can disturb the proper coordination of the front (incisal) teeth and the molars. In the maxillary dentition, the arch of the primary lateral teeth increases slightly in length, prior to being replaced by the permanent teeth. This helps the permanent lateral teeth to erupt properly between the incisors and molars. In the mandibular dentition, the length of the primary lateral arch decreases prior to its replacement by permanent teeth to enable the permanent lateral teeth to erupt into their correct positions (see Fig. 12 on page 82).

Relation Between Leeway Space and The Row of Lateral Teeth

The leeway space resulting from the different mesial-distal widths of the primary and permanent lateral teeth influences both the arrangement and eruption order of the permanent lateral teeth (see Figs. 11 and 12 on page 82).

Eruption Order Relationships In Lateral Teeth

The time of eruption for each of the lateral teeth is very close, from on tooth to the other, the eruption order of each tooth varies. Figure 12 shows the lateral arch in a case in which the eruption order of maxillary permanent lateral teeth was 4→4→5, and the permanent row was shorter than the final primary one. Each of these cases is normal and conducive to a proper arrangement of the permanent teeth.

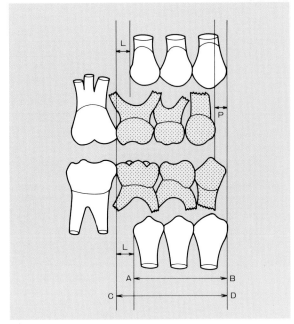

Fig. 11 Relation Between Crown Widths of Primary and Permanent Lateral Teeth. The difference (L) of CD and AB is called leeway space.

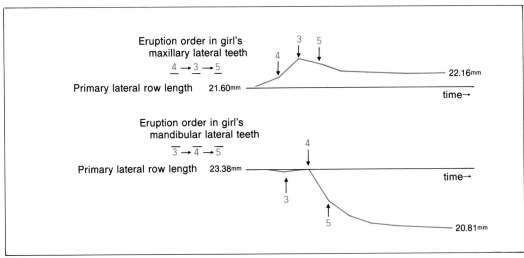

Fig. 12 Difference In Variation Patterns of Permanent Lateral Row Length Caused by Different Eruption Orders (4→3→5 and 3→4→5)

(Source: Hideo Iwata)

Summary

In observing the weekly progress of permanent tooth eruption for each type of permanent tooth, from the beginning of eruption to its completion, we have seen the different occlusal surface eruption periods and other differences that characterize the incisors, canines, and molars. Such factors as crown shape and the number of roots shorten the incisors' eruption periods and make molars' eruption periods four or five times longer.

The first molars stand out as having the largest and most complex occlusal surfaces and the greatest number of roots. Furthermore, their eruption period is also long, because of their function in lengthening the alveolar ridge by erupting on the distal side of the primary second molars.

The permanent second molars erupt on the distal side of the permanent first molars and also require a long eruption period. On the average, the maxillary first molars require 11 months for full eruption of the occlusal surfaces and the mandibular first molars require 17 months. The longer end of the distribution scale for first molar eruption periods for these teeth can vary widely from one individual to the next (see Table 1 and Figs. 32 and 33 on page 42). Full eruption of the permanent second molars requires on the average, 8 months for the maxillary teeth and 15 months for the mandibular teeth (see Table 2 on page 42).

The changes that occur in the gingiva between the start and end of eruption, vary according to the type of tooth. In the case of the molars, the gingiva recedes very slowly form the mesial to the distal sides, and this condition lends itself to the accumulation of plaque in the crown's grooves and sulci, as well as localized invitation of the marginal gingiva during the eruption process (eruption stages 2 and 3). In addition, there is a high incidence of caries during the eruption of first molars, and this risk is especially great during eruption stages 3 and 4.

Table 3. Eruption Periods of Occlusal Surface Eruption Stages In Various Permanent Teeth

Type of Teeth / Eruption Stage	Maxillary First Molar	Mandibular First Molar	Maxillary Second Molar	Mandibular Second Molar	Maxillary Central Incisor	Mandibular Central Incisor	Maxillary Lateral Incisor	Mandibular Lateral Incisor	Maxillary Canine	Mandibular Canine	Maxillary First Premolar	Mandibular First Premolar	Maxillary Second Premolar	Mandibular Second Premolar
	Weeks	Weeks	Weeks	Weeks	Weeks	Weeks	Weeks	Weeks	Weeks	Weeks	Weeks	Weeks	Weeks	Weeks
I	6	3	1	3	1	1	1	1	2	2	1	3	1	1
II	11	6	3	6	2	2	4	3	6	5	5	8	7	3
III	15	10	5	9	4	5	6	5	14	10	8	12	10	4
IV	20	20	26	20	5	6	9	6	15	12	23	15	14	6
V	28	22	29	22							25	16	15	7

Notes: (1) The numbers indicate the number of weeks since the start of eruption.
(2) The figures for incisors and molars are taken from the same example of eruption stages.

(Source: Sato Institute of Dental Research)

Results of Observations
Developmental Disturbances of the Permanent Teeth and Occlusion

Developmental disturbances are broadly divided into abnormal positioning, abnormal occlusion, and — related to these — abnormal number of teeth. Most of the causes for such disturbances are either hereditary, congenital, or in many cases, environmental. In addition, many cases of abnormal positioning of the teeth are caused by various conditions which occur during the replacement of primary teeth by permanent teeth.

1) Disturbances Affecting Particular Teeth

The results of a survey study conducted by Hisashi Saito, concerning cases of abnormal positioning of various teeth, showed such disturbances as diastema, crowding, twisting, and rotation occurring in 34.9% of the boys and 20.8% of the girls surveyed. These results showed that postnatal factors play an even bigger part in determining such disturbances than hereditary or congenital factors. Consequently, these results underscore the importance of tooth replacement for correct development of the alveolus (see Table 2 on page 85).

2) Abnormal Number of Teeth

Sometimes the eruption of permanent teeth is disturbed by an excess of teeth (supernumerary teeth) or a deficiency (missing teeth). Supernumerary teeth most often occur among the maxillary incisors and the mandibular premolars. Missing teeth most often occur among the maxillary second premolars and maxillary lateral incisors. Anatomical abnormalities occur most often in the maxillary lateral incisors and second molars and in the mandibular first and second premolars. In addition, there have been cases of a total congenital deficiency of teeth.

3) Abnormal Occlusion

In Hisashi Saito's study, mandibular mesial occlusion (reversed occlusion), mandibular distal occlusion (overbite), or reversed occlusion without mandibular mesial occlusion were found in 8.2% of the boys and 12.9% of the girls surveyed. When broken down into the three types of abnormal occlusion mentioned above, these were traced to hereditary causes in the great majority of individuals (all 8.2% of the boys and 7.9% of the girls), except for hereditary reversed occlusion without mandibular mesial occlusion, which occurred in only 5.0% of the girls.

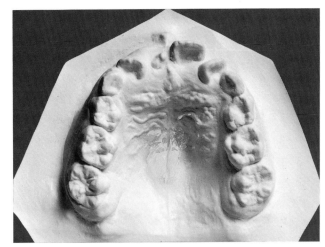

Fig. 16. Crowding of maxillary incisors (No. 10).

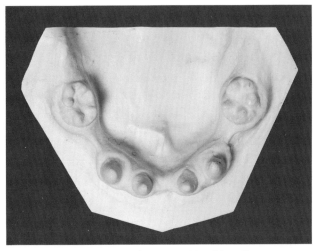

Fig. 17. Deficiency of mandibular dentition (No. 11).

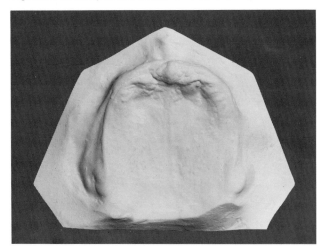

Fig. 18. Complete lack of maxillary dentition (8 years old) (No. 12).

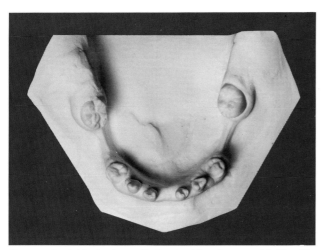

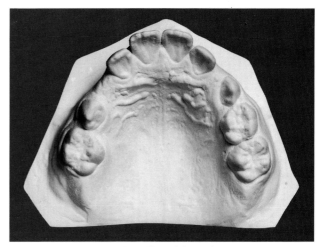

Fig. 19. Partial lack of mandibular dentition (8 years old) (No. 12).

Fig. 20. Transposition of maxillary right canine to second premolar position (Boy, age 11 years, 5 months) (No. 13).

Table 2. Frequency of Malocclusion in Primary Rows, Mixed Rows, and Permanent Rows of Teeth (based on 188 individual case studies).

Type of Occlusion	Primary Row		Mixed Row		Permanent Row	
	Boy	Girl	Boy	Girl	Boy	Girl
Normal	87.2%	83.2%	45.3%	51.5%	53.5%	65.3%
1. Diastema	1.2	2.0	4.7	3.0	2.3	1.0
2. Chaotic exfoliation	3.5	1.0	16.3	12.9	9.3	7.9
3. Twisting	4.7	4.0	23.3	13.9	19.8	8.9
4. Crossed occlusion	—	—	—	—	—	—
5. Open bite	1.2	4.0	—	3.0	—	1.0
6. Overbite	—	1.0	—	1.0	2.3	1.0
7. Protruding canines	—	—	—	1.0	1.2	2.0
8. Buck teeth	—	1.0	4.7	1.0	3.5	—
9. Reversed occlusion	1.2	2.0	1.2	5.0	—	5.0
II. Mandibular distal occlusion	1.2	2.0	4.7	7.9	7.0	6.9
III. Mandibular mesial occlusion	—	—	—	—	1.2	1.0

(Source: Hisashi Saito)

Comparison of Eruption Times for Permanent Teeth

The eruption of permanent teeth is influenced by overall body growth and development, and particularly by body height development. Variations in body height development have an influence on teeth eruption, as shown in a comparison of two studies — one conducted, in Japan, in 1955, and the other in 1982, in which eruption of the second molar occurred nearly a year earlier in the more recent study.

The rate of height increase during the ages of 5 to 8 ranges from 5 to almost 7 centimeters per year (see Table 3 on page 5). Table 1 shows a comparison of permanent tooth eruption ages, as surveyed in 1934 and from 1980 to 1985. The latter survey shows a relatively narrow age distribution, with eruption ages generally younger than in the former survey. There is thus a general trend toward earlier multiple eruption at certain ages. This comparison indicates overall that a trend toward a taller average height has accelerated the eruption ages of permanent teeth (see Table 1 and Figs. 1 to 14, on pp. 86 and 87).

Table 1. Comparison of Permanent Teeth Eruption Times (1934 and 1980~1985)

		Maxillary			Mandibular		
		Okamoto (1934)	Sato Dental Institute (1982)	Differential	Okamoto (1934)	Sato Dental Institute (1982)	Differential
Central incisors	Boy	7.66 years	7.11 years	0.55 years	6.75 years	6.33 years	0.42 years
	Girl	7.26	7.02	0.24	6.56	6.13	0.43
Lateral incisors	Boy	8.97	8.25	0.72	7.65	7.21	0.44
	Girl	8.44	7.97	0.47	7.40	6.95	0.45
Canines	Boy	10.99	10.69	0.30	10.38	10.04	0.34
	Girl	10.52	10.28	0.24	9.48	9.27	0.21
First premolars	Boy	9.89	10.06	−0.17	10.51	9.87	0.64
	Girl	9.55	10.01	−0.46	9.91	9.58	0.33
Second premolars	Boy	10.96	10.65	0.31	11.47	10.05	1.42
	Girl	10.67	10.57	0.10	10.87	10.34	0.53
First molars	Boy	6.77	6.59	0.18	6.38	6.29	0.09
	Girl	6.63	6.36	0.27	6.09	6.04	0.05
Second molars	Boy	13.01	11.91	1.10	12.28	11.55	0.73
	Girl	12.59	11.95	0.64	11.67	11.45	0.22

——— Okamoto
- - - - - Sato Dental Institu

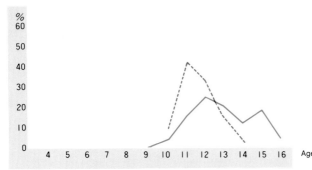

Fig. 1. Maxillary First Molars.

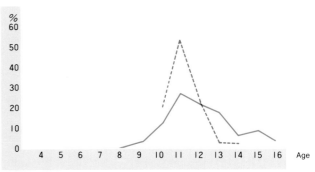

Fig. 2. Mandibular First Molars.

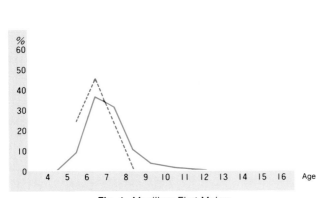

Fig. 3. Maxillary Central Incisors.

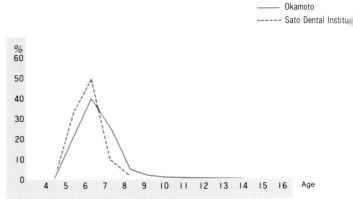

Fig. 4. Mandibular Central Incisors.

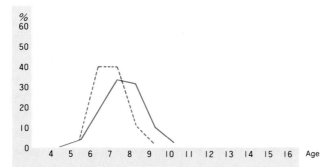

Fig. 5. Maxillary Lateral Incisors.

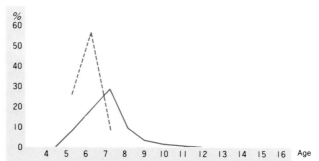

Fig. 6. Mandibular Lateral Incisors.

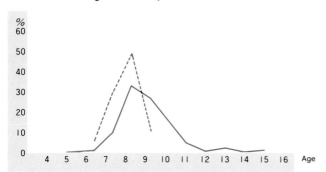

Fig. 7. Maxillary Canines.

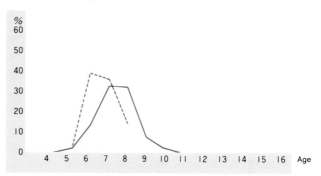

Fig. 8. Mandibular Canines.

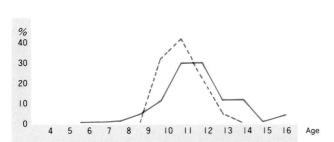

Fig. 9. Maxillary First Premolars.

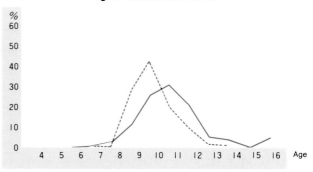

Fig. 10. Mandibular First Premolars.

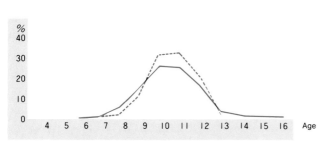

Fig. 11. Maxillary Second Premolars.

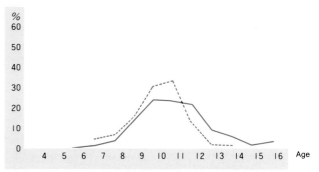

Fig. 12. Mandibular Second Premolars.

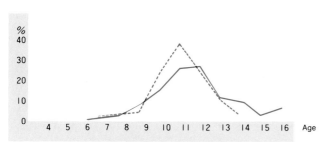

Fig. 13. Maxillary Second Molars.

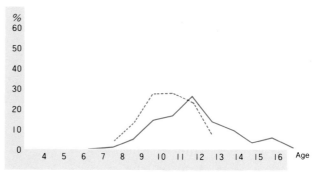

Fig. 14. Mandibular Second Molars.

Relationship of Caries in Primary Teeth to Caries in Permanent Teeth

Caries in the primary teeth is, characteristically, more rampant and progressive than in the permanent teeth. Caries occur most often in the maxillary and mandibular primary molars and the maxillary primary incisors, and less often in the maxillary and mandibular primary canines. It is especially frequent in the mandibular primary molars, during the ages of three to five.

When caries occurs in one tooth, it usually spreads to neighboring teeth, progresses rapidly, and can easily result in root infection. If the root has become infected, root resorption is often disturbed and the succeeding permanent teeth fail to erupt normally.

It is also common for caries, in primary second molars and in neighboring primary teeth, to spread to the permanent first molar, which then leads to problems in the entire permanent dental arch. Therefore, it is very important that measures be taken to protect the primary teeth from caries, thereby allowing the permanent teeth to develop and erupt normally.

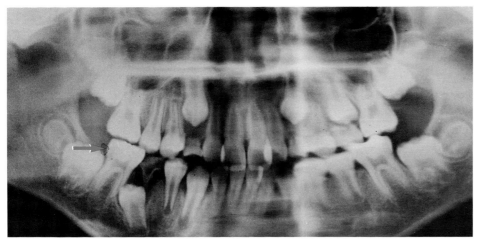

Fig. 25. Spread of caries from primary molar to permanent first molar (10 years, 6 months).

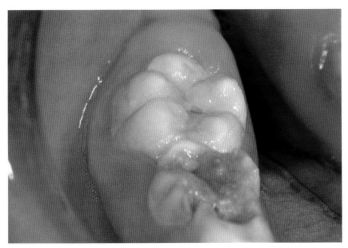

Fig. 26. Harm caused to permanent tooth eruption by caries in primary tooth (No. 206).

Radiographic Observation of Mixed Dentition

In pediatric dental clinics, X-rays should be used as an effective tool for illustrating such physiological phenomena as exfoliation of the primary teeth, the mixed dentition period, and the order of permanent tooth eruption. Concerning the relation between root resorption and succeeding teeth, radiographs are the only currently used method that allows the dentist to get a detailed picture of the extent to which permanent teeth have developed within the alveolus.

The mixed dentition period is also the time when the body undergoes a period of rapid growth and development. Normal dental development can be expected as long as the overall body's development is normal; however, any abnormality in this systemic environment can also affect dental development. Therefore, local variations, during the mixed dentition period, often do not remain local, but affect neighboring teeth as well and can even influence the development of the entire dental arch and its occlusion. It is therefore necessary, during dental examinations, to look out for possible adverse effects on future teeth.

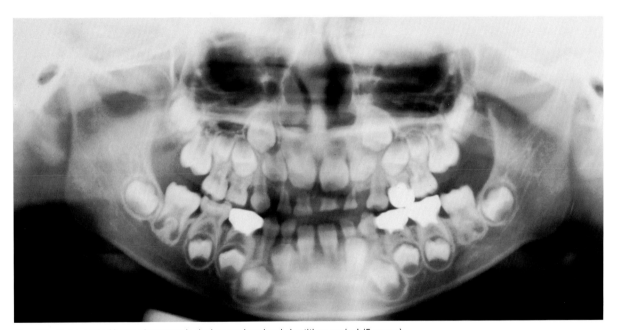

Fig. 15. Panoramic X-ray photograph during early mixed dentition period (5 years).

Caries in Permanent Teeth

(Particularly the First Molars)

Caries is a disease with many causal factors. It is known to occur very often on the occlusal surfaces of the first molars. The risk of caries is highest during the first two years after the eruption of the first molars (i.e. the first molars' first two years), which roughly corresponds to the one to three year period during which the first molars complete their eruption.

Survey studies revealed that, during the first 12 months after the first molars had started erupting, caries was found on 6% of the maxillary first molars and almost 20% of the mandibular first molars. During the first 24 months, this percentage jumped to 37% of maxillary first molars and 62% of mandibular first molars (see Table 3 and Figs. 28 and 29 on pages 90 and 91).

The four major types of caries causal factors are:
1. The susceptible tooth
2. Cariogenic bacteria in plaque
3. Substrates
4. Time (long-term accumulation of plaque, etc.)

In fact, caries is usually caused by a combination of some or all of the above types of causal factors (see Figs. 27 on page 90).

Let us briefly examine each of these four factors.

(1) Susceptible tooth: susceptibility to caries is largely determined by hereditary and environmental factors, and, in the first molars is also caused by such anatomical factors as the large occlusal surface and the numerous deep sulci, grooves and fissures. In addition, a long period is required for eruption and, during this period, the tooth substance is still young.

(2) Cariogenic bacteria are also part of oral microbiota. It is considered that they cause infection by proliferating together with other many kinds of microbes. Cariogenic bacteria known to the present time are Streptococcus mutans, Streptococcus sanguis, Lactobacillus lactis, Actinomyces viscosus and Actinomyces naeslundii.

(3) Substrate (glucides): adherence of plaque to teeth is a natural consequence of the teeth's role in eating. Glucides are a likely base substance for bacteria, and especially fermentable glucides, such as saccharose, which make up a conducive environment for the outbreak of caries.

(4) Time: two temporal factors combine to contribute to tooth decay. These are (1) the time since eruption in which the teeth lay exposed in the mouth, and (2) the period of time that elapses before the plaque is removed.

Therefore, the environment most conducive to rapid outbreak of caries is that found during the first molars' eruption period.

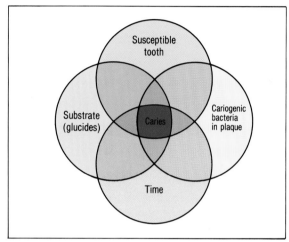

Fig. 27. Environmental causes of caries.

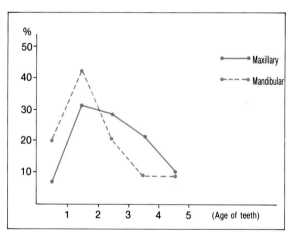

Fig. 28. Annual rate of caries occurrence during first molars' first five years. (Sato Institute of Dental Research)

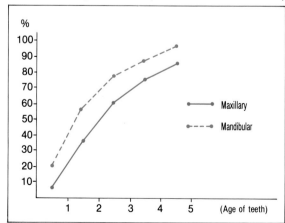

Fig. 29. Accumulative rate of caries occurrence during first molars' first five years. (Sato Institute of Dental Research)

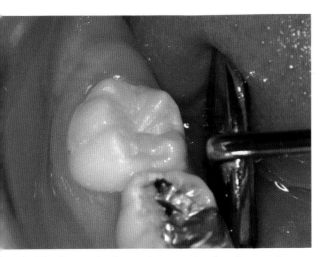

Fig. 30. The first molar has a large occlusal surface and many grooves (No. 207).

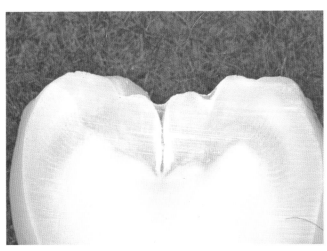

Fig. 31. Plaque can easily accumulate inside the central fissure and grooves (No. 14).

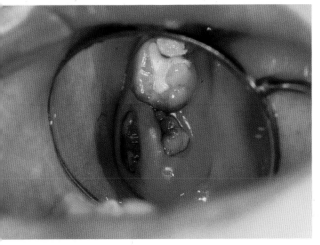

Fig. 32. The first molar is easily contaminated during its eruption period. This photo was taken during the 12th week of eruption (Page 13, Fig. 12).

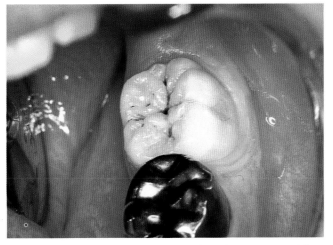

Fig. 33. Caries has broken out, starting from the grooves and fissures (No. 208).

Table 3. Rate of caries occurrence in first molars.

Age of teeth	0	1	2	3	4
Maxillary (No. of teeth checked)	194	166	111	52	21
Annual Rate of Caries Occurrence	6.2%	30.7%	27.9%	21.2%	9.5%
Accumulative Rate of Caries Occurrence	6.2	36.9	64.8	86.0	95.5

Mandibular (No. of teeth checked)	202	178	124	77	35
Annual Rate of Caries Occurrence	19.3%	42.3%	19.4%	7.3%	8.6%
Accumulative Rate of Caries Occurrence	19.3	61.6	81.0	88.3	96.9

(Sato Institute of Dental Research)

Prevention of Dental Caries

To find the most effective means of preventing dental caries, we must ask ourselves how best to prevent caries during the period in which it is most likely to occur. As mentioned earlier, this period of highest risk is the first two years following the start of the first molar eruption (see Table 3, page 91). During this period, the first molars are still young and have not yet fully matured, which means they have a low resistance to decay. This factor, makes it a period during which there is no naturally occurring inhibitor to caries infection.

Within the high-risk period, the most dangerous time is during eruption stage 3 (about 15 weeks after the start of eruption). During this period, the occlusal surface is strongly contaminated and difficult to clean. This remains the case for the entire one to two years required for full eruption to the occlusal line. Focusing upon this highest-risk period, let us consider the following five methods for prevention of caries.

1. It is nearly impossible to brush the first molar during its first 12 weeks of eruption. Therefore, fluoride should be applied and the child's parents advised of proper eating and brushing habits (eruption stages 1, 2, and 3).
2. At about the 13th week of eruption, the central fissure appears above the gingiva. At this point, direct preventive measures such as fissure sealants, can be applied (eruption stage 4, see Figs. 30 and 31, on page 92).
3. At about the 15th week of eruption, brushing becomes possible. However, ordinary toothbrushes (Fig. 33, page 93) will not work, since the tooth has yet to reach the occlusal line. Therefore, a special molar brush should be used (eruption stages 4 and 5, see Figs. 32 and 33, on page 93).

4. Fig. 35 shows the results of tests using an ordinary brush and a molar brush, (Fig. 33, page 93) for repeated brushing. As can be seen in the figure, the molar brush proved to be a more effective cleaning tool (see Fig. 35 on page 93).
5. One final preventive tool is a broad and correct awareness of the oral environmental conditions, age, lifestyle, and dental hygiene attitude of the patient, particularly during the period in which direct preventive measures are advisable — namely, the period between the beginning and end of first molar eruption.

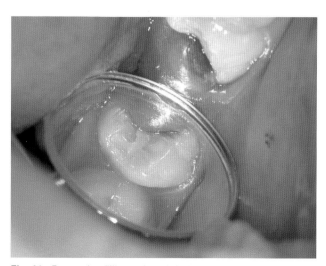

Fig. 30. Preventive fillings placed during eruption stages 2 and 3 (No. 209).

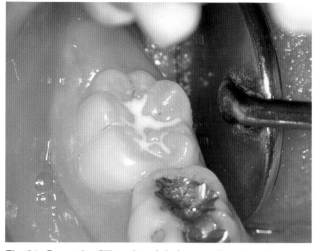

Fig. 31. Preventive filling placed during eruption stage 4 (No. 210).

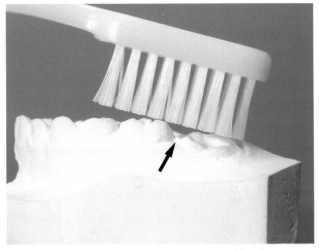

Fig. 32. During first molar eruption, ordinary toothbrushes cannot clean the tooth thoroughly (No. 15).

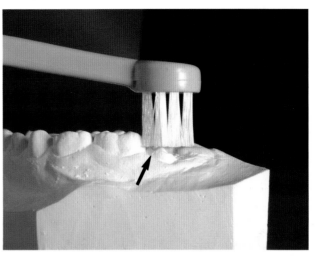

Fig. 33. Special molar brushes are able to clean the entire occlusal surface (No. 16).

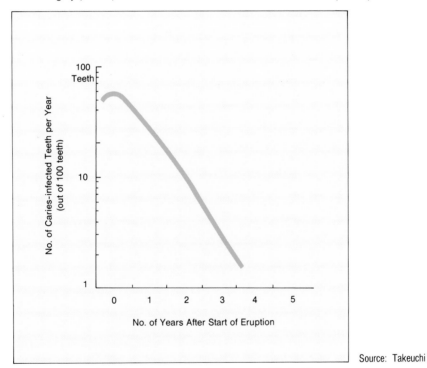

Source: Takeuchi

Fig. 34. Number of first molars infected with caries during each of the first five years of eruption (subjects were children who each ate approximately 20 kg of sugar per year).

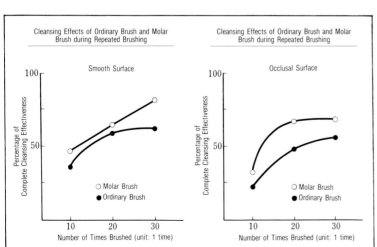

Source: Lion Dental Hygiene Laboratory

Fig. 35. Comparison of cleansing effects of ordinary brush and molar brush during repeated brushing.

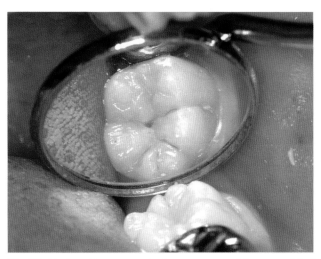

Fig. 36. Caries often occurs in the grooves and fissures of first molars (No. 211).

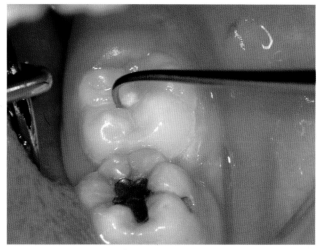

Fig. 37. Use of explorer to diagnose early caries (No. 212).

Caries Activity and Food

It is a well-known fact that some types of food are more conductive to caries infection than others. There has also been epidemiological evidence of a positive relation between the occurrence of caries and the amount of sugar consumed. Mitsuharu Takeuchi has demonstrated a strong correlation between these two phenomena, and has shown that the influences of sugar intake on teeth is especially strong during the first years following their eruption. (See Fig. 34 on page 93)

B.G. Bibby et al. have reported on the variation in caries occurrence produced by several different types of suctose-containing foods. In addition, Takashi Matsukubo et al. have produced a table listing several types of food and such caries-conducive characteristics as "plaque forming ability". (PFA), "acid producing ability" (APA), "intake time" (IT) and "coating time" (CT). These

studies all underscore the importance of choosing the proper foods for children and restricting their intake of sweets as a preventive measure against caries. (See Table 4 on page 95)

Table 4. Foods that Easily Lead to Caries Infection.

Substantial Characteristics		Temporal Characteristics		Food
PFA	APA	IT	CT (after swallowing)	
HIGH	HIGH	MEDIUM	HIGH	Toffee, Caramel, Nougat
HIGH	HIGH	HIGH	LOW	Candy, Lollipops (hard candy), gum
HIGH	HIGH	LOW	HIGH	Wafers, Sweet-bean filled rice cakes, Angel food cake, Chocolate biscuits, Sweet beans, Biscuit cookies
			MEDIUM	Sweet-bean filled buns, Chocolate, Fired caramel dough, Cookies
HIGH	HIGH	LOW	LOW	Thick malt syrup, Cakes, Jam, Sweet flavored gelatin
MEDIUM	MEDIUM	LOW	LOW	Vanilla ice cream
LOW	LOW	LOW	HIGH or MEDIUM	Potato chips, Rice crackers, Shrimp chips, Sorbitol chocolate, and Cookies made with coupling sugar

Source: Matsukubo

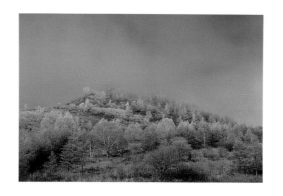

REFERENCES

1) Aizawa, K.: Roentgenological study on growth of the permanent teeth. *Kagoshima Igaku Zasshi*, 33: 206–219, 1960.

2) Ariga, K.: Relation between eruption of the right upper lateral incisor and growth in sitting height. *Jap. J. Dent. Health*, 7: 125–135, 1958.

3) Atkinson, Spencer R.: Growth and Development of the Teeth (A) Mandible (B) Maxilla. *AM. J. Orthod.*, 26(8): 29–84, 1940.

4) Baume, L. J.: Physiological tooth migration and its significance for the development of occlusion (I) The biogenetic course of the deciduous dentition. *J. Dent. Res.*, 29: 123–132, 1950.

5) Baume, L. J.: Physiological tooth migration and its significance for the development of occlusion (II) The biogenesis of the accessional dentition. *J. Dent. Res.*, 29: 331–337, 1950.

6) Bibby, B. G., *et al.*: Evaluation of caries-producing potentialities of various foodstuffs. *J.A.D.A.*, 42: 491–509, 1951.

7) Carr, L. M., *et al.*: Eruption ages of permanent teeth. *Austral. dent. J.*, 7: 367–373, 1962.

8) Cohen, J. T.: The dates of eruption of the permanent teeth in a group of Minneapolis children, A preliminary report. *J. Amer. dent. Ass.*, 15: 2337–2341, 1928.

9) Danae, Apostlides talmers: The times of eruption of second permanent (12 year) molar and its relation to body size and sexual maturation. *Am. J. Phys. Anthrop.*, 10(2): 262, 1952.

10) Friel, S.: The development of ideal occlusion of the gum pads and the teeth. *Amer. J. Orthod.*, 40: 196–227, 1954.

11) Fukada, H. *et al.*: Abnormal root resorption of deciduous teeth. *Skikageppo*, 29: 103, 1955.

12) Fulton, J. T. and Price, B: Longitudinal data on eruption and attack of the permanent teeth. *J. dent. Res.*, 33: 65–79, 1954.

13) Halikis, S. E.: The variation in eruption of permanent teeth and loss of deciduous teeth in Western Australian children. IV. Sequence of permanent tooth eruption and deciduous tooth loss. *Austal. dent. J.*, 7: 400–408, 1962.

14) Hellman, M.: Nutrition, growth and dentition. *Dent. Cosmos*, 65: 34–49, 1923.

15) Hellman, M.: The process of dentition and its effect on occlusion. *Dent. Cosmos*, 65: 1329–1344, 1923.

16) Hurme, V. D.: Ranges of normalcy in the eruption of permanent teeth. *J. Dent. Child*, 16: 11, 1949.

17) Iwasawa, T.: Relationship between sequence of exchage of intact dentition and malocclusion. (Part 1) Sequence of exchange of intact dentition. *J. Jap. Orthod. Soc.*, 18: 125–147, 1959.

18) Kamijo, Y., Sato, K., Haga, T. and Shimura, O.: The study on the eruption of permanent teeth. (Part 1) Age changes of the erupted state observed by eruption type. *Shikwa Gakuho*, 52: 333–335, 1952.

19) Kaneda, A., Inada, M., Kanemitsu, A., Ito, M. and Watanabe, S.: Statistical observation for yearly changes of dentition of permanent teeth on the pupils in junior high school. *J. Osaka. Odontol.*, 22: 1448–1452, 1959.

20) Kitamura, H.: Biostatistical study on eruption order of permanent teeth. *Bull. Tokyo Dental Coll.*, 9(1): 1–28, 1967.

21) Kitamura, S.: Untersuchung uber die Durchbruchsdaten und die Reihenfolge der bleibenden Zahne. *Shikawa Gakuho*, 41: 191–198, 1936.

22) Kitamura, S.: Studies on time and order of eruption (I). *Shikwa Gakuho*, 47: 274–287, 1942.

23) Kitamura, S.: Studies on time and order of eruption (II). *Shikawa Gakuho*, 47: 352–368, 1942.

24) Kunimoto, A.: A study on statistics of dental caries (I). *Jap. J. Dent. Health*, 6: 4–23, 1956.

25) Logan, W. H. G. and Kronfeld, R.: Development of the human jaws and surrounding structures from birth to the age of fifteen years. *J. Amer. dent. Ass.*, 20: 379–427, 1933.

26) Lo, R. T. and Moyers, R. E.: Studies in the etiology and prevention of malocclusion (I) The sequence of eruption of the permanent dentition. *Amer. J. Ortho.*, 39: 460–467, 1950.

27) Lo, R. T. and Moyers, R. E.: Studies in the etiology and prevention of malocclusion (I) The sequence of eruption of the permanent dentition. *Amer. J. Orthod.*, 39: 460, 1953.

28) Lysell, L., Magnusson, B. und Thilander, B.: Time and order of eruption of the primary teeth. *Odont. Revy*, 13: 217–234, 1962.

29) Matsui, S.: Studies on relation between eruption of permanent teeth and body growth. *J. Jap. Dent. Ass.*, 13: 1–11, 1961.

30) Moorrees, C. F. A.: The dentition of the growing child, a longitudinal study of dental development between 3 and 18 yeras of age. Harvard University Press, 1959.

31) Moyers, R.E.: Handbook of orthodontics (3rd ed). Year book Med. Publ., 1973.

32) Nance, H. N.: The limitation on orthodontic treatment (I) Mixed dentition diagnosis and treatment. *Amer. J. Orthod. and Oral Surg.*, 33: 177–223, 1947.

33) Ogiwara, Y.: Biostatistic study of the eruption order of deciduous teeth. *Bull. Tokyo Dent. Coll.*, 12(1): 45–76, 1971.

34) Ohta, H.: A Biostatistic Study on Falling Out of Deciduous Teeth and Eruption of Permanent Teeth. *Shikwa Gakuho*, 66(10): 1016–1049, 1966.

35) Ohta, H.: Biostatistic analysis of the shedding of

REFERENCES

deciduous teeth and the eruption of permanent teeth. *Bull. Tokyo Dent. Coll.*, 8(2): 95–122, 1967.

36) Okamoto, K.: Variative statistical study on the dates of eruption of permanent teeth. *Shikwa Gakuho*, 39: 139–170, 1934.

37) Okuya, K.: Study on the period and the order of eruption of permanent teeth. *Shikwa Gakuho*, 7: 30–38, 1950.

38) Orban, B.: Growth and Movement of the Tooth Germs and Teeth, *J.A.D.A.*, 15(16): 1004–1016, 1928.

39) Osanai, H.: Study on Yearly Transition of Eruption of Permanent Teeth of Pupils in Aomori District. *Shikwa Gakuho*, 59(9): 689–710, 1959.

40) Saito, K.: Correlations in the Times of Eruption of the Lateral Teeth between the Upper and Lower Jaws. *Shikwa Gakuho*, 70(12): 1581–1589, 1970.

41) Saito, K.: Statistical Study of Correlations between Eruption Times of the Upper and Lower Permanent Teeth. *Shikwa Gakuho*, 70(12): 1590–1608, 1970.

42) Sato, H.: The types of eruption and their development during the beginning of mixed dentition. *J. Stomat.*, 28: 204–217, 1961.

43) Sato, S.: Studies on the growth of teeth in Japanese. (I) Seasonal fluctuation of the eruption of permanent teeth. *Medicine and Biology*, 47(5): 183–187, 1958.

44) Sato, S.: Studien uber das wachstum der zahne der japaner jahreszeitliche Schwankung beim Durchbruch derbleibenden zahne. *Der Offentliche Gesundheitsdienst*, 22: 86–89, 1960.

45) Schour, I. and M. Massler: Studies in Tooth Development of the Growth Pattern of Human Teeth. *J.A.D.A.*, 27(12): 1178–1798, 1940.

46) Shinomiya, S.: Studies of relationship between permanent teeth eruption and menoplania. *Jap. J. Dent. Health*, 9(3): 257–267, 1959.

47) Sicher, H.: Tooth Eruption, Axial Movement of continuously growing Teeth. *J. Dent. Res.*, 21(2): 201–225, 1942.

48) Sicher, H.: Axial Movement of Teeth with Limited Growth. *J. Dent. Res.*, 21(4): 395–402, 1942.

49) Steggerda, M. and Hill, T. J.: Eruption time of teeth among Whites, Negroes, and Indians. *Amer. J. Orthod. and Oral Surg.*, 28: 361–370, 1942.

50) Stones, H. H. *et al.*: Time of eruption of permanent teeth and time of shedding of deciduous teeth. *Brit. dent. J.*, 90: 1–7, 1951.

51) Tanaka, T.: Climatic effect upon the eruption of permanent teeth. *Niigata, Med. J.*, 73(1): 93–102, 1959.

52) Yanagisono, Y.: Relation body growth and eruption of permanent teeth. (Report 2) *Kagoshima Igaku Zasshi*, 33: 299–314, 1960.

53) Yoshimi, M.: Statistical studies on the period of eruption of permanent teeth. (Report 1) Observation on the discontinuous sample of children in Hirosaki in 1949. *Hirosaki med. J.*, 7: 235–241, 1956.

Japanese references are omitted in this English edition.

INDEX

ABOUT THE AUTHOR:

Dr. Sadakatsu Sato, *D.D.S., D.Med.Sc.*

Born in 1917 in Fukushima Prefecture, Japan.

In 1943 graduated from Tokyo Dental College.

Since 1949 head of Sato Institute of Dental Research.

1949～1954 advanced studies in hygienics at the Medical Department of Keio University.

1954 received the doctorate degree (D.M.Sc.) from Keio University.

Since 1954 instructor in oral hygiene at Tokyo Dental College.

Since 1967 part-time instructor at the dental hygienists' school attached to the School of Dentistry, Tokyo Medical and Dental University.

1978～1981 Chairman of the Japanese Society of Dental Practice Administration.

1980～1989 Japanese representative on the board of directors at the international headquarters of the International College of Dentists.

In 1990 President of the above international organization.

Dr. Sato is also the coauthor of the
Textbook of Dental Practice Administration.